# FROM THE HEART

# FROM
## THE
# HEART

## A MEMOIR AND A MEDITATION
## ON A VITAL ORGAN

## JEFFREY L. KOSKY

Columbia University Press   *New York*

Support for the publication of this book was provided by the Class of 1956 Provost's Faculty Development Endowment at Washington and Lee University.

Columbia University Press
*Publishers Since 1893*
New York   Chichester, West Sussex

Library of Congress Cataloging-in-Publication Data
Names: Kosky, Jeffrey L., author.
Title: From the heart : a memoir and a meditation on a vital organ / Jeffrey L. Kosky.
Description: New York : Columbia University Press, [2024] | Includes bibliographical references.
Identifiers: LCCN 2024024925 (print) | LCCN 2024024926 (ebook) | ISBN 9780231217644 (hardback) | ISBN 9780231217651 (trade paperback) | ISBN 9780231561839 (ebook)
Subjects: LCSH: Meditation. | Contemplation. | Philosophers.
Classification: LCC BL627 .K68 2024  (print) | LCC BL627  (ebook) | DDC 158.1/2—dc23/eng20240927

Cover design: Julia Kushnirsky
Cover image: Shutterstock

*To*
*Marsha and Michael Kosky,*
*Claire and Oscar Kosky,*
*and*
*Stephanie Hodde,*
*with gratitude and appreciation*

# CONTENTS

**PART II** HAVING A HEART IS
A CHRONIC CONDITION

# PREFACE

*March 2024.*

It often appears the world is conspiring against those who want to have a heart. A country, my country, at war with itself. An international order that is crumbling, a planet that is collapsing. Teen suicide rates. Punishing assessment regimes govern life, the lives of young people especially. Failure is not an option: ongoing assessment and ever-rising metrics assure we don't. Time always seems to be running out, in my day, for my homework, for the planet, and so on.

Heartlessness might be the safest option, a logical conclusion.

This book avoids reaching that conclusion. It comes from the heart. While not blind or deaf to heartrending matters of global, political, and social concern, in it I speak more personally and meditate on life and death matters out of the experience of having a heart, the one I call mine.

That experience has not been easy.

In the summer of 2018 I learned what it feels like to have a heart when I lost it. I was clearly dispirited. Most of the summer was spent indoors, avoiding projects that concerned me, refusing friends who called on me, and in general hiding from the day by staying in bed. I slept a lot—two naps before the end of my workday as a scholar and teacher, then frequently another before dinner. Dispirited, I didn't have the heart for anything. Then, one afternoon, I felt it fail. It missed a beat, many times. I felt dizzy, and the world flickered off then on, off then on. The moments it darkened were fleeting, as fleeting as the beat of a heart—as the missed beat of a failing heart, that is. When the world came back on again, nothing had changed. But everything was different. And nothing would be the same again.

Hastily scheduled visits to the doctors as well as advanced imaging procedures confirmed that my heart was failing. I was fifty years old. This shouldn't have been happening. My aortic valve was not closing properly, and my heart was struggling to pump against the significant volume of blood flowing backstream. Something as small as the aortic valve of my heart had stopped functioning correctly, and my days vanished: meaningful projects were over before they had come to an end, things I cherished were dropped, and most of my loves proved unattainable. I was falling out of the world. My life hung in the balance, and it was swinging unsteadily.

Cardiac surgery repaired my heart. My aortic valve was replaced. The balance in which my life hung steadied, but that was not the end. As much as I would like to say that the story ended with the success of cardiac surgery, there remained the return to the days of daily life, and that is not easy. How do you explain to others where you have been when you stood close to the threshold of death? How do you deal with everyday concerns such as deciding which toothpaste to buy when you had to decide for surgery that involved stopping your heart and sawing through your breastbone? How do you imagine giving your time to sitting through a committee meeting when you cannot forget the fact that your whole life, your entire being, your heart, can fail and be lost, a fact you know to be true because it happened? It can be very difficult to share the apparent concern others have for choosing toothpaste, attending meetings, or shopping for a new couch when your to-do list still has on it "Don't die." My priorities were different, and so too my sense of security. Nothing had changed when I returned, yet everything was different. It was bewildering.

It still is bewildering. My loves all seem very fragile now, the loss that comes with their possession an ever-present shadow of their enjoyment. The valves don't last forever, and I now live with expiration dates on my heart. There will be another surgery. My life still hangs in the balance.

In my bewilderment I am learning many lessons, seeing many things that become visible only in the darkness. Having a heart to lose means confronting big questions. Those questions are my meditations on living and dying with a heart I call mine. When I lost it, I found myself in a position to reflect on what it feels like to have one. This book is where I did that. In writing it, I have come to believe strongly that we should listen carefully to those who find themselves at a loss, ill or diseased, weak or vulnerable, impoverished or unabled. Not only to honor them and let them have a voice, but because they offer valuable data for understanding what it means to inhabit the chronic condition of our human being. Anecdotal evidence, to be sure, but in this book I try to listen to the one closest to me, the one more intimate to me than even myself: my heart; and in listening to it, speak from it, from the heart.

The bulk of this book was written in the two years or so following my diagnosis. Those years included the failure of my defective heart; the decision for surgery and the subsequent surgery itself; then what is often known as recovery, the return to everyday life. This last I am finding to be a still ongoing process: the circle of homecoming, it turns out, is one that doesn't close, for the point of departure to which one goes back is never the same again. Many of the pages were written in the midst of the events they describe. The resulting book tries to remain faithful to that sometimes overwhelming experience of not knowing what was going on while trying to find the heart to go on anyway. It includes passages from journals alongside pages written more formally. Some of the pages concern my encounter with works of art and literature; others reckon with medicine and medical history. Making sense of what is happening calls for both reckonings. My world, all my loves, all my projects and concerns, depend on the effectiveness of modern medicine. Its history is mine, thanks to the decision we made to commit to cardiac surgery. Understanding what is happening to me must therefore take account of that history, which I do in this book. But, although it can repair the heart, modern medicine did not give me the heart I need to get on with everyday life. I still had to find, still have to find, the heart to return to the days that cardiac surgery gave me. That, too, is what I do in this book. In the end, *From the Heart* weaves together philosophy, religion, literature, and the arts with a personal narrative told in the context of medicine and medical history to reflect on matters of life and death, the "big questions" I confront when I found, when I find, I have a heart to lose—something you, too, can say.

# FROM THE HEART

# THE BEGINNING

## It's Hard to Have a Heart

*August 26, 2018.*

It's hard to have a heart these days. Much about our society is cold and severe. It does to the heart what the artist Jeff Koons does to it in his work *Hanging Heart*: makes it hard and steely, all surface and impenetrable. You can see it in an image made by Emmanuel Dunand.

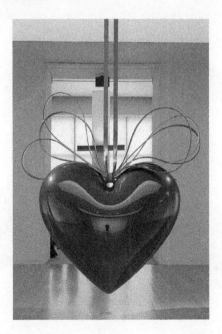

Hearts like this won't get crushed, the perfect thing for a difficult and challenging world where, we are told, success demands focus and shrewd calculations.

A steel heart that is nevertheless pretty.

It often appears Koons is right about our hearts: you must hang yours, until it is dead, or leave it hung out to dry if you want to succeed in life. We all know this, don't we? The young people I meet in the university classroom do. They know very well that it takes a steely heart to make the harsh decisions demanded by daily life in a world where every threat is also an opportunity for those with an entrepreneurial spirit. At the very least you must steel your heart, let it grow hard and impenetrable, to maximize advantage without cracking under pressure or even just growing faint from all the exertion.

When a cold and heartless society does treat matters of the heart, it makes that heart bright red and shiny, tied up in a bow for easy consumption, like you see in this image made by Hubert Fanthomme: a rendezvous with Jeff Koons's *Sacred Heart*.

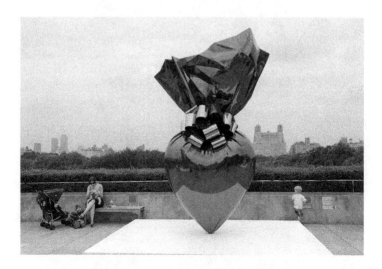

He is right again, unfortunately: the sacred moments of a society in which we hang our hearts look and feel very much like this. If sacred time is, as a common definition holds, time that is "wholly other" than the time of profane everyday life, if it is time "set apart" for activities that are other than those that make up the business of life, break time, as it were, then it should come as no surprise to hear that our sacred time is devoted to glamorous vacations or wild intoxications, adventurous excursions or dreamed-of dropouts in the spa—all of which are packaged, ready-made, and easily produced en masse, even when expensive. Reflecting ourselves and our reality back to us in splendid forms, brilliantly colored and dazzling, *Sacred Heart* is emblematic of the feel-good aesthetic for which Koons is known. "I just try to do work that makes people feel good about themselves, their history, their potential," he says, and who, in a society that hangs its hearts until they are cold and steel, if not stone, wouldn't like to have a heart bright red and shiny tied up neatly in a bow, packaged and ready-made for easy consumption. "I believe that my journey has been to remove my own anxiety," he continues. "The more anxiety you can remove, the more free you are to make that gesture. . . . If the anxiety is removed, everything is so close, everything is available."[1] When anxiety is desperately avoided, matters of the heart are made easy to deal with, and having one can only be pleasurable, gleeful—fun, in short. Following your heart, we are led to believe, is the secret to a life of bliss, and the path followed straight and smooth. Hearts never seem heavy.

The world in which anxiety is desperately avoided, it bears repeating, is the hardhearted world in which you steel your heart for the business of life, life become a business to succeed or fail at. That heartless world of the *Hanging Heart* is the world for which the heart is never heavy, never darkened by anxiety but always bright red and shiny, the same world that makes the *Sacred Heart*, so shiny and easy to possess.

It is an odd world we have come to where hearts are hard enough that they never break yet are always light.

My own heart is heavy to bear and easily lost. That was a lesson that came crashing over me undeniably this summer, 2018. It was a difficult time for me. I am usually able to get out of bed early, before my wife and children, an ability that is especially important in the summer months when everybody, being either a teacher or a student, is at home and a few precious morning hours starting at 5:30 or earlier are the most reliable times of peace for writing and reading. This also has the advantage of freeing longer hours of the day for work on our place or time spent with family. But this summer I struggled to rise before 8:00, frequently failed at that, and then often found myself napping again before 11:00. It had always been typical for me to lie down to rest in the early afternoon, around the lunch hour or shortly thereafter, usually for twenty or thirty minutes; it can be invigorating and refreshing. Those rests became sleeps this summer, the pause that refreshes the slumber that never ends. They stretched to sixty then ninety minutes, even a full two hours, and when I woke, I rose groggy, still cloudy. As for working our place, I am usually energized by it. The property is not large, about 3.25 acres, but it is also not small for someone who came here from urban Chicago and had never before ridden a lawn tractor, cleaned a gutter, or tended a garden. There is a lot to do, especially in spring and summer when all that there is to do comes on very quickly, tasks being called for in rapid succession. I can usually rise, slower than needed but still rise to the challenge until the swelter of July and August keeps me inside, but this summer I retired before the middle of May and ignored the weeds that needed to be pulled in favor of hours inside mostly sleeping or reading fiction. The vegetable garden grew grass knee-high; paths I opened two summers ago behind the old barn closed again; poison ivy returned on a hillside that past diligence had nearly eradicated. The edging having been neglected, the place was becoming shapeless again.

I was clearly losing heart. My spirits were low, and my courage was failing as I grew deaf, nonresponsive to the world in which I might have found myself had I been able to look. Lying in bed for long hours, resting, with the door shut so the children would not see me in my weakness (as if they did not already know), or else sitting in a club chair in the cool of my bedroom, looking without focus, I ignored the claim exerted on me by the yard and any thing or person calling. Dispirited, I was, as I said, losing heart.

It turns out I was right in more ways than I knew. One morning, sitting at my desk, reading and writing and enjoying the freedom of it, my heart skipped a beat, several beats or a beat several times, really. Putting my fingers to my neck to take my pulse, I found signs of the heart I was losing. I felt six normal beats then nothing, six normal beats then nothing, and so on again and again for maybe ten cycles. During those intervals of nothing, it was as if the world blinked or the filmstrip of consciousness's stream had had a few frames snipped out, instants of blackness that change nothing but make everything tremble. Everything remained in place, but nothing was the same. I was lightheaded, faint, and dizzy, so I went upstairs to lie down and rested until, thirty minutes later and still a little dizzy, I called the doctor for an appointment. After seeing my primary care physician the next day, then, by some blessing of good luck, my cardiologist the day after, blood work and, more significantly, an echocardiogram, we knew it was indeed my heart that was

defective: an insufficiency of my aortic valve meant that a significant amount of blood was flowing back into the left ventricle of
my heart with each beat, causing the muscle to work harder
with each pulse to counteract what the experts call "severe regurgitation." The weakness and fatigue, as well as the throbbing in
my head and surging in my chest, were explainable by this.

I was indeed losing heart: the organ was defective and now
defecting from the rest of me. In fact, it is not much of an organ
if it is neither an effective means to an end nor an instrument that
serves its master. My heart was defecting: it was not obeying my
command that it deliver more strength, more power, more vitality; it was inefficient and not helping me produce more effects in
the world I wanted to make for myself. My heart was defecting—
as if it were not really mine—and the defector threatened to tear
me apart.

It's hard to have a heart.

We decided on aortic valve replacement surgery and soon after
set a date, September 18, 2018. Perhaps then my heart could be
mine again? Perhaps then the heart would be a mere organ again?
That is, it seems, the operative premise of medicine in the minds
of many who practice and partake of it, and it is a good one, one
that I gladly endorse and one I assumed in choosing to undergo
the surgery that would replace my defector, the valve I had had
from birth, with one that would do my bidding and thereby let
me live longer and better. They said I would be better than ever,
that I might not even recognize myself with my newfound energy.
Having had this defect from birth, I have after all never known
what it is like to have a heart that functioned effectively as an
organ. I could be whole, me all the way through myself.

These were some of the reasons we gave as we rationalized our
decision. They were some of the hopes we entertained as we

looked ahead in expectation of the future we imagined. But in the irrepressible background of these hopes and reasons lurked a set of questions that remained troublesome and pressing to me, metaphysically inclined as I am. Even if the hopes are realized, the expectations come to pass, and the reasons prove justified, will it be I who am better; will it be the same I who is "cured" as the one who needed help? What does "cured" mean? At what point do we say recovery is over and I am recovered? Maybe even more important, do I want the cure if it means I won't recognize myself afterward? Yes, I do, but what does that say about who I am not the same as myself? These are not unrelated to questions of importance to religion, revolving as they do around the issue of beginning again, being reborn, and being made "whole." I should therefore know something about them, professor of religion that I am, and yet those questions and their answers signified anew and in new ways for my now very concerned questioning. This is not even to mention the one big, obvious question that shadowed the expectations that made up our days: What if it doesn't work? What if they put me in a coma, cut me open, and can't put me back together again?

My defect was congenital, a bicuspid rather than tricuspid aortic valve. This defect can also be acquired, usually in early childhood when a rheumatic fever results in scar tissue that damages one of the three leaflets composing a fully functional aortic valve. Mine was detected just before high school. Few restrictions were placed on me, and I competed in sports and other activities like most kids my age. I had to see a cardiologist annually who used imaging technologies to track the progress of my heart's defection. These were noninvasive, in fact the same technology used to provide images of a fetus in the womb of a pregnant mother, and over the years they grew more and more sophisticated, easier to administer, and more detailed in what they gave us to see. Many people with this defect are asymptomatic or have symptoms so mild, an unusual rush in the chest, an occasional fullness that makes you catch your breath, that they go through everyday life blissfully unaware of the defect at heart. These are the happy people—who might one day find their defect has become a total failure, heart failure, a failure of the heart whose left ventricle has enlarged through overexertion in countering the excessive regurgitation, grown stiff, and then slowly loses, irrecoverably, the strength to go on, until eventually the heart they have easily and blissfully forgotten is finally lost forever.

I am, as I said, lucky not to be one of the blissful. My defect was detected when I was in high school. My good luck meant I lived knowing this day would come, knowing that one day they would saw open my breastbone, stop my heart, cut out the old valve, and sew in a new one. Good luck.

In the meantime, until that day arrived, I lived with the background awareness that it was indeed good luck that I needed since bad luck meant the day arriving before its time. With this possibility hanging over me at every moment, good luck let me continue on. For the most part there were very few reminders of this fact. I experienced few limitations from my condition, and none of the doctors I saw placed overly inhibitive restrictions on me: I shouldn't lift the neighbor's car out of a ditch; I shouldn't practice powerlifting; and I shouldn't forget to take the pills, calcium channel blockers commonly prescribed for high blood pressure, coronary artery disease, and abnormal heart rhythms, that would defer and delay my day of reckoning by relaxing blood vessels so that my defector could pump more easily and therefore longer. Without too many real possibilities restricted from me, the reality of my heart's defection did not impose its presence insistently and should have been easy to forget in everyday life.

And it was, for the most part. As with much of individual-ization and growing up, repressing and suppressing existential truths that touch intimately at the heart of who we are proved essential to living everyday life and its happiness. Neglecting these, living in their oblivion, I could be one of the happy people. After the teenager's initial shock at hearing his future lifesaving surgery laid out before him by a gray-haired man wearing a lab coat, I went about my business absorbed in life and the happiness of living it, with only the occasional reminder of an annual visit to the cardiologist making me aware of my good luck.

Until this summer, when my birth finally caught up with me or I with it. The heartbreaking summer of staring at our clear-ing in the forest through my bedroom window, of listening only half-aware to the stories my son would tell of new feats on the trampoline—this heartbreak showed me the truth of my birth, vaguely sensed and dimly intuited all my life but now undeni-able. I had to face it, face up to the truth of my birth. This heart has been defective ever since I was. It never worked the way I wanted it to. I have always been worried about death. I have always been inhibited in action and decision. I have always flinched before overexertion outdoors and wanted to stay inside while the other kids played hard and sweated. I could forget that or neglect the truth of what I have been from birth and did so happily—until my heart's defection became complete and it no longer served, did not do the work I asked it to do realizing my intentions to get here or there, to lift this or that, to be present attentively to him or her before me. Its defection was never entire, never that bad; good luck meant we caught it before then. But I now see disclosed the truth that I was never fully in command, never fully possessed of myself—that having a heart means liv-ing with this defect.

It's hard to have a heart.

Compare Koons's *Hanging Heart* to that of Mark C. Taylor in *Homage to Jeff Koons*.

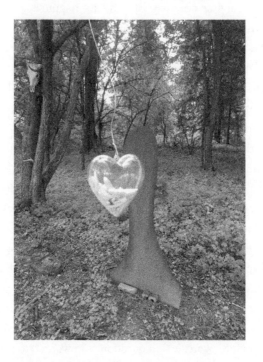

Taylor hangs his heart not on his sleeve in a high-profile, glamorous location where all can see how shiny it is but more discreetly from a tree in a dim grove found in his place on Stone Hill in the mountains outside Williamstown, Massachusetts. The hanging tree grows in the boneyard he cultivates there, a small grove of trees alongside the drive that connects his house to the forested road and eventually the state route that leads back to town. The trees appear to grow skeletons: skulls, femur, clavicles, pelvises and so on from deer, cow, buffalo, and other once living animals whose bones are nailed to the trees. The grove sits on a slowly rising incline, it is shaded and dark, making it difficult for one's look to penetrate all the way through. There does not appear to be a light at the end of the tunnel, yet in the shadows of the place all around you, you sense a luminosity, a luminous darkness glowing without visible source. It is a place apart, a sacred grove, the perfect place for Taylor to hang his hearts.

The boneyard is part of a larger installation, a sculpture garden Taylor has been tending for more than twenty years. The sculpture is formed of rocks and bones unearthed in his exploration of the place that has made up his life since he arrived there in 1989: thrusts of ledge rock, a stream from an underground source, matters like this discovered in the process of clearing the land to hold open the field where Taylor finds his life's work now shaping up.

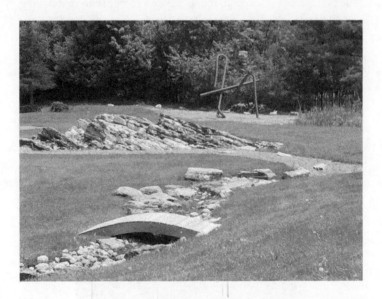

It is no exaggeration to say that Taylor has put his heart into this place. Why? Why hang your heart here, in this remote place that calls for so much time, effort, and money? He knows that such questions have no answers. He calls the garden a "folly" and writes, "No Romantic ruins. There are, however, pyramids, though they are flawed—broken and inverted. . . . Somehow, things just got out of control. Hours, days, weeks, years of unproductive labor. And for what?"[2] Follow your heart and it ends up like that: out of control, unproductive labor, *Wozu?*, to what end, *à quoi bon?*—what remains are bones, like those that fill Taylor's hearts. We can lie to the youth (the college kids I meet in my classrooms) and tell them otherwise: we can tell them that following your heart is the sure path to bliss or to success, that having a heart makes life as happy as having a birthday present or carnival prize tied up in bows every day, but then we are selling them a cheap and ultimately heartless version of the heart. More heartfelt and true to the facts, it seems to me, is Taylor's recognition that having put all his heart into it, this work, a true vocation, like all labors of love, is "beginning to seem more my undoing than my doing."

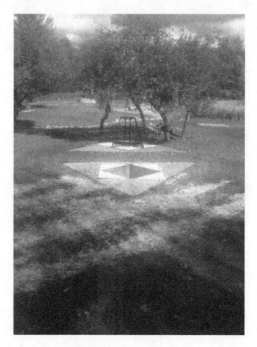

Some will take the boneyard to be evidence of a morbid obsession and despairing anticipation of death, but that is far from the case: the place is living evidence of vitality, Taylor's and that running through Stone Hill. There is a pulse, Taylor senses, beating in the place. He attends to it and carefully shapes it into the work that emerges from the ground. Forms have grown from rock and stone, a stream flows from an underground source, and trees weep, of all varieties, where before there were none. Taylor's work is obviously vital, vital to all that, but where does his vitality come from?

Is it work that comes from the heart? It's certainly not an entrepreneurial spirit that undertakes such losing plans, and it's not the spirit of an administrator. If he is the founder, owner, and manager of an art factory (and he does manage a lot of stone-workers, backhoe operators, welders and casters, and so on), he has a lot to learn from Jeff Koons about the steely heart required for success. The books just don't balance in this work of the heart. He has sunk a lot of time and money into the place, time and money that will never be recouped. The real estate agents have already told him as much, but work that comes from the heart comes from elsewhere than the office of the salesman or the desk of the accountant.

If Taylor's heart is activated by his sensitivity to Stone Hill, steeling his heart against the place would surely mean a diminishment of vitality. He works in the boneyard, then, not so as to earn what it takes (wages) to be free and independent (eventually a boss or manager and then retiree), nor does he work so as to close himself securely against the givens of the place, its clemencies and inclemencies, the vagaries of the weather, and so on. Rather, his work opens him to the place, and the place to him. "This place has become a part of my life, and I have become a part of its life," he writes. When this happens, when the hands of place and the hands of self shake, the life he senses pulsing through Stone Hill circulates through him, too, as if it were the case that when he is sensitive and feels the beating of the place, it beats in him as well. "The earth moves me as much as I move it" is also how he puts it.

This sensitivity to the place makes for a surprising heartiness. Just look at the forms he has brought to light. "It is no longer clear where body ends and earth begins," he finds, when he is, for instance, raking rocks and pebbles into the patterns of wash from the stream. The work emerges there, with the double binding (and I am reminded that religion as *re-ligare*, according to one possible etymology, means to bind again) of body and earth, his life and the life of the place that pulses through him. This double binding, this religion, Taylor names "nexus" and, following the philosopher Maurice Merleau-Ponty, *chiasmus*, a double enfolding, interlacing or implication that is a coimplication of each in the other.

We could also call it *heart*, if we listen to the medievals who thought about the heart before its modern picture as a pump was drawn up by William Harvey (1578–1657) and his heirs. The historian Heather Webb has collected numerous accounts from them: medieval poets, natural philosophers, theologians, and scientists, too, who tell of a heart that is porous and in its porosity resembles Taylor's *nexus*.[3]

Whereas the heart we moderns have inherited from Harvey is a pump in a closed system of intrabodily circulation, the medieval heart is more like a room or, perhaps better, passage where traffic and mixing takes place with others and things of the world. Bodies out there, the medievals say, have a presence or aura that is real in spirits exhaled naturally just by their very being. These spirits are welcomed, inhaled, into the heart that resides in me, the heart being in this way my vulnerability to the presence of others and things. Memorable examples come from Dante and from his colleague and mentor Guido Cavalcanti, both suffering the presence of their loves. Speaking of his unnamed beloved, Cavalcanti exclaims, "Love pulled sighs from your eyes, / shooting them into my heart so strongly / that I fled, confounded." What circulates through the poet's heart, then, is not just his own blood. Passing through his heart are also breathed sighs, the sighed spirits pouring from the eyes of another who looks upon him. His heart senses them, and he is moved, in this case to run away. Consider also Dante, who suffers the spirits that "fly from the beloved's eyes" and enter his heart before he knows it. "I felt the beginnings of an earthquake in my heart, as if I was in the presence of this lady . . . and then I saw the wondrous Beatrice approaching," he exclaims. This sensitive, fragile young man is touched by the presence of another before he has put up his guard. That touching presence is sensed, before something is seen, in the heart—which welcomes those spirits, no matter how confounding or how shaken I might be by the earthquake they trigger.

The open heart is also a warm heart, and together warmth and openness make for vitality, as the medievals explain. The welcoming heart warms the spirits it receives, mixing them with blood and humors inside us to produce something new, the "little spirits." These are diffused through my body via arteries, animating it, inspiring me, as it were, in what would be my otherwise dispirited state. Open and warm, porous, the medieval heart, then, is where we are bound chiasmically in and with things and others, a nexus, as Taylor puts it, neither fully mine nor fully another's. This nexus proves vital and vitalizing, inspiring because place of inspiration. One loses spirit when this nexus, heart, is lost.

From a warm and welcoming heart come inspired works, Webb's medievals go on to tell us. How so? The spirits inspired from bodies and things outside are warmed in the heart to such a degree that they rise, like all volatile spirits, and are lifted, high spirits, to the point that they press or are breathed out, expired or expressed, vibrantly in the world, taking form in the emotions and the actions that make up our everyday, but also in the more exceptional forms given them by the poets whose hearts, inspired by the spirits of others, expire or breathe out elevated spirits in the form of words, that is, poems. Their poetry is a heartfelt work, their words often carried by its sighing spirits or tears.

These examples remind me: hearts of stone, impervious, cannot receive the spirits vital to mine; and a cold heart does not have what it takes for that vitalizing transformation. No wonder Dante depicted the bottom of Hell as a frozen lake, not a fiery furnace, in which the most wretched lives were stuck, encased up to the neck with hearts of stone buried in the ice. These are the traitors, the ones who willfully cut themselves off from traffic with others and their spirits. There is and will be no heart-to-heart with a traitor, no spirited exchange with such a betrayer. With the heart in their chest sunk in Hell's pool of ice, frozen solid and stony, no words of song are breathed out from their mouth, not even a sigh that would fly up to heaven like that of Dante when his heart was struck by the spirits flying from the gaze of his beloved, Beatrice. Only "chattering teeth" (32.36). Even worse, these icy hearts are not warm enough to stop the tears from freezing in their eyes before they can be shed—a fate discovered in Brother Alberigo, who begs visitors to his Hell to "remove the stony veils from my face, / So that the grief can issue from my heart / A little, before the tears freeze up again" (33.112–14). In Hell, where we are cursed to actually and finally get what we want, forever, the coldhearted find they cry but shed no tears, cannot, in other words, shed the tears they cry now and forever. Unshed, the tears freeze in their eyes and make an icy mask that steels them, like Brother Alberigo, against the world. Imagine that: crying whose work of shedding is frustrated; nothing issues from it, crying that becomes fruitless as well as isolating, isolating in its fruitlessness, fruitless in its isolation; a crying in which grief does not cry out and circulate but stagnates. These cold hearts, these hearts of stone, were hearts steeled against the outside. Now they are cold hearts, hearts of stone, hearts steeled against the outside—getting what they want: to be sealed into the inside.

Tears flow from a warm heart, and if I let my heart be warmed by "the spirits that fly from the beloved's eyes," I might cry. I surely do when I imagine saying goodbye to Stephanie and Claire and Oscar on the day I know will arrive when I will be wheeled into the operating room. A soft heart won't last forever like a stone one might: it melts. Taylor sees and knows this. It's why there are bones at the heart of his work. I see those bones in my heart of hearts, too. They are coming.

If it is right to say that Taylor puts his heart into Stone Hill, it is also the case, I think, that he finds his heart there, too. That heart is one he feared he lost in a life-threatening crisis several years previously, one narrated in his book *Field Notes from Elsewhere*. Stone Hill is for him, it is no exaggeration to say, the place of recovery—in the several senses of *recovery*. Taylor writes about this recovery in a book suggestively titled *Recovering Place*. It is not just about a return to or rediscovery of place and its importance, finding what was lost; it is also about the place of recovery, the place where recovery in the sense of "healing" happens. In Taylor's case, that recovery is organized around the crisis of septic shock following an infection and then the ensuing discovery and treatment of a cancer. His case is different from mine, then, in that he experienced a crisis, I am subject to a condition. Whereas he had to recover from a disease that nearly killed him, I will have to recover, they say, from the surgery that will keep me from being killed. It involves stopping my heart and sawing open my sternum, major trauma from which I will have to recover—at least, I hope to have the chance for recovery.

Taylor's life-transforming events are recounted in his earlier book *Field Notes From Elsewhere*. I take *Recovering Place* to be the continuation of the story of recovery that began in *Field Notes*, but by no means does Taylor's recovery story end in a supposed completion on Stone Hill. It remains ongoing, chronic in this sense, more like a condition. As he writes, "even when the diagnosis is good, full recovery remains an idle dream. The problem is not to find a cure, but to learn to live with the impossibility of cure."[4] What, then, do they mean when they say my recovery will be six to eight weeks? When the impossibility of a cure becomes the condition one must learn to live with, recovery, Taylor tells us, or learning to live anew, means learning to die: "I am beginning to realize that I returned to Stone Hill to learn how to die and, by learning how to die, learn how to live anew."[5] The place of recovery is marked by heavy hearts, laden as they are with the bones to which life clings.

Recovery has long been recognized as the work of the sacred. Rub the sacred stones on wounds, and they heal. Drink from the sacred chalice, and life is hale. Find the sacred grove, and you are healed from the suffering of what has been lost. But, if the sacred heals, Taylor's sacred heart nevertheless holds skeletons.

The sacred that makes whole (heals, hale) makes hale by admitting to life the bones it includes. Recovery of life brings thoughts of death. Though vigorous, Taylor's heart is filled with intimations of its eventual breakdown, failure: bones. When you look at this heart, you do not see a shiny image of yourself. This heart does not flatter in that way. Instead, when you look into this recovered heart, what you see is bones, skeletons.

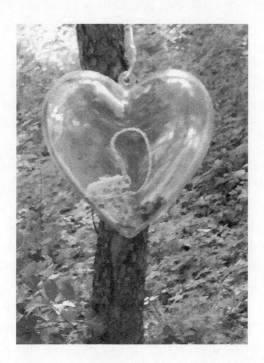

Where Koons makes hearts with shiny, impenetrable surfaces that protect us from seeing that inside, Taylor makes hearts that admit being looked into, but the skeletons you see when you look into them are not what you want to see. These hearts are full. Their fullness come from the end they intimate. For those who think life is a carnival, a shiny red heart tied up with a bow is the perfect one to have; but for those who sense there is more to life, such hearts ring hollow. Life's hard knocks sounding on a steely heart will eventually prove as much. Taylor's heart is weighty to be sure, whereas Koons's is light and seems almost to levitate, but that is because the latter's shiny, steel heart is empty, filled only with hot air, whereas Taylor's is full, filled with the bones on which living flesh hangs. Looking into Koons's *Sacred Heart* you see reflections of yourself in the cold, steely surface of the world. Looking into Taylor's, you see what remains, what remains when the idols of self-reflection have been smashed and are broken.

Bearing the bones of the living, these hearts are not easy to take up. "People die in your heart," says the artist Karen Green, widow of the author David Foster Wallace. She knows that what is held in a heart dies, turns to fleshless bone. Exposure to that is what it means to have a heart. Keeping others near and dear, having them at heart, means keeping this loss near and dear, always, always with them. Hearts are not hollow and are not meant to be empty, or if they are, it is the empty hollowness of a container. In this void that they are, they are meant to contain something, something that is bones eventually.

Green's poetic remark is the other side of the consoling truth "he will live in your heart," a truth we commonly hear from others and one we imagine her having heard frequently after Wallace's death. When thoughts of his loss come over her, Green initially entertains this comforting thought but cuts it short: "he will live in your,"[6] for she knows that what is held near and dear in the heart is the loss that defines all the others we know and love. That is inevitable when the container is defined by being open, like a heart.

All hearts will defect, then, mine and those of the others I hold close to me by holding them in mine. Taylor reminds me of that. It is as if he shows me their brokenness as a special because definitive possibility, a possibility that is definitive of the heart's very being. A broken heart is not so much the end in which the heart disappears and stops being itself but the possibility that defines it as a heart.

I lived for the most part and most of the time in a healthy denial or oblivion of that definitive possibility, but now I have come to know it undeniably, as my heart's defect has become insistent during these months of incapacity, lassitude and irregular, out of control pulses coursing through me.

What is the worry? At times when the throbbing in my head is great or when my breath taken away by the surge welling up in my chest—in those times, I might worry about getting to the surgery, but the doctors never really do. When I think about the surgical procedure itself, splitting my sternum, cutting into my heart to cut out the old valve, stitching in a new one (cauterizing it? No, they don't do that, the doctors assure me), then, yes, I do worry, but again the surgeon doesn't. While "routine heart surgery" is probably an oxymoron to the layman, the procedure itself has proven fairly low-risk and the technique seems standardized, almost automatic. There are surgeons who have performed thousands of them now, making for a cult of experts that did not exist at the time my defect was first detected, and my surgeon, though only fifty-four years old, has been in the business for twenty years or so. As I said, the experts never seem particularly worried about the surgery or my getting there, so I put my confidence in them: they have the numbers on their side (less than 2 percent complication rate), and there is comfort in becoming just a number, just one of the many who have already had the procedure; the anxiety will go away.

But that's hard to do, I am finding, when your heart is at issue.

Having decided on the critical care of my heart, what will be the outcome of this medical intervention? Sure, complication rates are 2 percent or less, but am I one of the 98 percent? Having chosen to take up the burden of my defective heart with this intervention, what sort of life will we be making? What if I feel the same after the intervention? Is that still success? It might work, but it might not. In the case that concerned me, mine, it might not work for me. I could be one of the 2 percent. Having decided to fight, which side will be victorious, I wondered—like the Christian Saint Augustine in his *Confessions*, where he gives voice to his own anxiety about the heart that he takes up in the act of conversion.

Augustine knew well that the heart is a weighty matter. Having one, he finds, means I am "a burden to myself," as he puts it. He speaks this confession from the position of mortal creature, given over to the constitutively defective yet good condition of human being in all its weakness and incapacity. When matters of the heart are taken up in confessing them, it is in unknowing ignorance, he says, of how these matters will turn out: joys and sorrows are at war and "on which side the victory lies, I do not know" (10.28). The uncertainty of the outcome arises not simply because external obstacles threaten finding, getting, and keeping the heart whose home he believes he knows. It is not just that we are powerless to decide the outcome even when we have our heart set on it. It is also and perhaps even more so the case that having a heart means he is unable to be decisive in deciding and controlling where it lies, where to find it and where to put it. "Our hearts are restless," he confesses in the opening page. They are the place where opposites contend and we vacillate, hesitate, and waver. Unquiet or restless,

I therefore become when I take up matters of the heart, my heart. This makes for the trial of life.

This is not an easy place to be. Believe me. Weak and ignorant, unable to give himself the power he needs to be in charge of winning or losing the trial of the life he faces when he has a heart, Augustine finds himself dependent on the graces of another and cries out, "Have pity on me, O Lord in my misery." Wretched, then, is the position of the confession in which he takes up his heart—not simply because it means being there where he doesn't know on which side the victory lies, but also because it puts him in a position where the source of the power that makes all the difference is not one over which he is master. I will soon put mine in the hands of the doctors and already, I confess, find my heart given over to my wife, my children, my students, and countless others whose inspired spirits are ingredient to determining mine.

Deciding to deal with the matter of my heart by committing to the lifesaving surgical procedure, we were not so much released from as given over to the worry of a life concerned about itself and the quality of its involvement in the world. My wife heard from colleagues whose spouses had had valve replacements that we would hardly recognize me, I would be a new me, born again, as it were, my first birth erased and with it the defect that was congenital. This thought, I suspect, is an illusion fulfilling the dream of redemption from the condition of birth, a religious dream perhaps but also the dream of those who idolize Jeff Koons and his *Sacred Heart*. Believers both sides. The truth is that even the plastic valves, the mechanical ones that replace the defective ones we have from birth, have expiration dates: studies show they survive somewhere around fifteen to twenty years before they too need replacing. Clearly, then, even the best outcome would mean continued worry. Happiness once reached brings with it the worry of keeping it. If there was to be a rebirth, a new me, it would not be the only one. If I was going to be born again, I would have to face up to the disappointing fact of that birth and having to be born again and again.

Taking up the problem of having a heart means living on with its eventual failure. Not taking up that problem means heart failure will no longer be an ongoing possibility but a realized reality as it were. Deciding for the life-giving surgical procedure, then, brings with it the worry of having a heart. If the surgery does not worry, the life it will give me does.

I started to measure it out, in terms of expiration dates. Surgery now in 2018 at age fifty meant another at age seventy, when the life of a replacement valve expired. Then another at age ninety, after another term had expired? Probably not, for if the risk of surgery on a seventy-year-old man was already significantly greater, it could be catastrophic for a ninety-year-old man. Conclusion: I will not live past ninety. Not a bad limit, but a limit nonetheless, one that three of my four grandparents did in fact surpass. My days are numbered. But perhaps we could recalculate, run the numbers differently so that I could survive two replacements: do it now at fifty, then again at sixty-five, regardless of my condition at the time, so that the third could be done at eighty, then I might make it to ninety-five. My grandparents lived into their mid-nineties, after all. I should be able to do that, too. There was yet another way to look at the numbers. Given that mortality rates ten to fifteen years following surgery rise dramatically when the surgery is done on older patients, then a surgery at sixty-five still looks promising, the next surgery at eighty less so. Maybe then one should do the second surgery at seventy so as to have a good chance of making it to eighty-five. But one's chance of making it to seventy after a valve replacement at fifty is not as great as one's chance of making it to sixty-five, and doing it at sixty-five gives a good chance of making it to eighty but less likely to make it to eighty-five. So while replacing it at sixty-five seems to make the next replacement fall on a better schedule for reaching the possibility of ninety-five (because you might get another replacement in at eighty), replacing it at seventy might make it more likely you reach eighty-five. Which do you choose?

The numbers never lie, but there are lots of ways you can count them. Is it madness to have ever started?

From now on, my heart will be stamped indelibly with an expiration date. It's a fact that I will be living with expiration dates. These days there is enough data available that those who know and can count can calculate with some reliability the odds, not the certainty, of my making it to such and such a date. Up to a certain age, I can probably take comfort in the numbers they give me, but there will come a turning point when the odds are against me.

When you begin calculations regarding matters of the heart, about the only thing that becomes clear, if you are honest with yourself, is that your days are numbered—and then, numbered, you count them more and more. In the best of all worlds, they, the days, would count more and more, but it is a sad truth that most of the time I counted them, making them count less and less, in an endless worried calculation that never consoled the worry it intended to cure. Meant to maximize the utility of my heart and thereby secure the optimal outcome for myself, these were in fact cold calculations, treating matters of the heart more like commodities with a shelf life. They were ways to steel myself against the uncertainty of victory and "I know not what" that Augustine said was inevitable when life took matters to heart, really to heart. They were making my heart a *Hanging Heart*, hanged and already dead in life.

Against that calculative logic, there must be another logic.
The logic of the heart?

The surgery itself involves stopping my heart. That's hard for me
to say, very hard: they will stop my heart. It's a terrifying thought.
After they stop my heart, they will hold it still while they cut. I
will be in their hands, literally and entirely. Good luck. I will be
handing over my heart entirely to the hands of an other, others
in fact: surgeon who cuts my heart, anesthesiologist who stops
it, intern or resident who opens my chest, and so on, not to mention all the others—nurses, friends, family—who will be with
me in the days, weeks, maybe months of recovery and rehabilitation. Having a defective heart, and aren't they all defective,
short-lived or shorter-lived than any of us would like, I have to
give it over to these others in order to have it. If I keep mine, I
lose, it and everything.

They will cut out the valve I was born with and stitch in a new
one. You can see it in the picture. One like it sits in a package
on a shelf in the hospital, available for the next one who needs
it—that one being these days not just anyone but me.

They will also cut out a segment of my ascending aorta. It has
an aneurysm that makes it thin and weak. They will replace it
with a tube made of Dacron, a material used in fishing lines,
clothing, and firehoses. Without these, I will not live, at least not
very much longer. Autonomous and independent? Hardly. My
body is my own, a site of integrity? Not really. Not only do I need
that artificial valve inside me, that mechanism stitched to my
organism with seams that can hardly be seen but are there, but
I need all the knowledge and expertise, all the technology and
design, that is the context in which such a tiny device is possible. A hundred years ago, I would be dead or at least have very

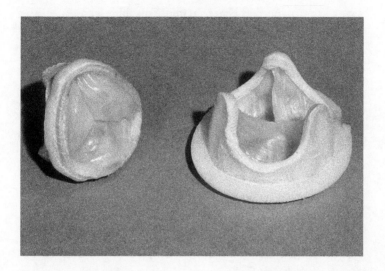

little life left. Fifty years ago and I might make it, but the odds
would still be against me.

But they won't just stop my heart. For some stretch of time,
they will replace it with a machine, and my blood will pulse to
another's beat. That too is a terrifying thought. Doesn't some of
the terror come from the prospect of becoming heartless in this
way: they will stop my heart and put in place a pump, nearly
autonomous that beats on its own, unstoppably it would seem,
perhaps forever, but without me. A heart of steel. Can I be
replaced so easily? My heart is a machine. It is dehumanizing and
depersonalizing, I fear, and reduces all this anxious writing in
search of a meaning or a meaningfulness to it all, reduces it to
insignificance if the heart is just a pump, a mechanism made to
operate again by plumbers. What's the concern? Why worry? Of
course, that way of looking at it is precisely what makes it possible for it to succeed. To the surgeons, I have to imagine, I don't

have a heart so much as I have a pump, a machine whose mechanical operation they can know and predict and therefore design and execute surgical interventions that will ensure its more efficient and prolonged operation. Thank God for that.

But still, I am at issue in this business. It's not just a heartless matter. They will hold my heart in their hands, and it will beat to their tune. The anticipation is obviously troubling. Can I find the heart to go on with this matter of my heart? Mine is failing.

Seen another way, only a heart undergoes heart failure and finds itself at a loss. Listening to it means listening to what one day will stop.

The artist Dario Robleto listened carefully to a heart, his grandmother's, as she lay on her deathbed. He tells a moving story of having had the opportunity to hear the last beat, the last five beats, in fact, of his grandmother's heart when he laid his head on her chest to hear her speak what would be her last words.[7] The beats grew steadily farther apart, the lapse between each elevation in her pulse growing longer, the moment of rising from each fall more and more delayed. Ear to her chest, he waited attentively, hanging himself devotedly on the ebb and flow of blood pulsing through her body, a pulse powered by a heart over which he had no control. The life in her beating on at its own pace and its own rhythm, for its own time—not knowing how long that would be. One can only imagine how much heart it took for him to wait attentively for the next beat of hers, each growing farther from the previous, each arrival demanding more and more patience and deference to its slow coming. Each moment of his time stretched out to the measure of her beats.

Which beat is the last?

This is the problem of course with every "last," every "last one" or "last time:" you don't know when it is, only when it was. You don't know until you have passed beyond it, and even then, might it still be a matter of waiting just a bit longer? Having heart means never knowing which beat will be the last, until after it is when you no longer can. In that sense, those with a heart always miss the full significance of the moment, realizing it too late because late to the end. In the present, being attuned to the heart that beats in life throws you into attentive waiting, holding your breath, as it were, until the next beat. You might die waiting.

This is not despair talking. This is sensitivity to the heart and its matters. The despair is instead the hastiness that waits no more, deciding to make this one the last regardless by leaving and getting back to business. Sometimes despair might be warranted. Robleto did not despair, however, of the heart's fragility, its ultimate weakness, unable to go on. He waited. He had the heart to wait long enough to wait for the next, not knowing when the last would come, and waited longer each time.

But it came. It always will. There comes a moment when the waiting is over. For every heart, there will have been a last beat—without a present in which it is noted, experienced, and made mine. When Robleto admits that the last has come and gone, the waiting turns into memory, sadly a memory of what it does not hear—the beating of the heart.

As Robleto tells it, it *was* a great privilege to tune in to that pulse as it died, a moment of almost unspeakable intimacy from which he was obviously energized and moved to make the moving work of art he makes. It *is* a great privilege in other words to have a memory of what he does not hear. That privilege is memorialized in an art installation by Robleto that I saw, and more amazingly heard, at the Massachusetts Museum of Contemporary Art, MassMOCA, in summer of 2016, the year I also saw the hearts hanging in Mark Taylor's boneyard. It is work that comes from the heart, the chiasmic heart-to-heart with his grandmother on her deathbed. Titled *The Boundary of Life is Quietly Crossed: An Unknown History of the Human Heartbeat*, it documents a history of the human heartbeat from early attempts to transcribe a pulse to the fabrication of an artificial heart.

The first time "the inner workings of a still beating human heart" were seen in a situation of everyday life—without surgical incisions or violence, that is—was when the German physiologist Karl Vierordt recorded the pulse of his beloved wife, Pauline. That was in 1854. Motivated by the desire to, as Robleto puts it, "know, hear, or feel the other's heart," Vierordt constructed a device that Robleto describes as similar to today's blood pressure device: a pulsing artery activated a lever attached to a human hair, the finest most responsive "stylus" Vierordt could imagine, that inscribed lines in soot pooled on a strip of paper that moved beneath the hair. We still have the picture of that pulse. Using it, Robleto reverse-engineered the sound such a pulse might make so as to let us eavesdrop on the spirits that circulated between these two lovers' hearts, the one whose pulse we see (Pauline's) and the one whose pulse it aroused (Karl's), or else also, chiasmically, the one aroused by his ministrations (Pauline's) and the one attentive to hers (Karl's).

Equally fascinating to listen to is Robleto's reanimation of the first recorded fetal heartbeat, a recording made in 1908. The chief problem, as he tells it, is one of sensitivity: finding a device that is sensitive enough to register "life in its first eager beats" while it is sheltered in the womb. The first practicable solution to this problem of sensitivity was that of Otto Weiss. It involved detecting "the tiny vibrations of the fetal heartbeat *by use of a soap bubble*, a membrane of such delicacy that it far exceeded any microphone of the era." A soap bubble! A bubble of soap serving as a drum skin beat by the vibrations of air produced by the pulse of life in a fetus. "To record this action," Robleto tells us, "Weiss

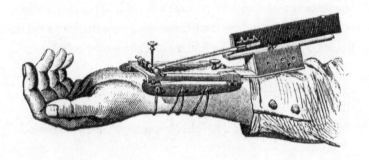

placed a silvered glass thread, thinner than a single hair, at a right angle inside the bubble with one end of the glass thread attached to a holder to keep it in position. . . . As the soap film's membrane absorbed the sound waves and beat in unison with the heartbeat, it transferred its movements to the glass thread, and like a pebble tossed in a pond, the thread absorbed the ripples into its form. . . . Focused light [entered] the device, projected onto the rippling glass thread. The casted shadow of this thread was then projected onto photosensitive paper producing a photograph of the movements of the undulating line."[8]

Pictures traced by a human hair dangling in "the residue of a candle flame that burned in the 19th century"; photographic images of shadows cast by a thread of glass so fine it could be moved by a soap bubble—these are the effects of a beating heart. They are the work of the heart. Epoch-making they are not: history takes little notice of a heartbeat. Shiny and glamorous, hardly: this work does not do much to call attention to itself. This is what comes from the heart. It is the most quiet of forces, with ever so slight and fragile an effect. It takes an almost unbelievable sensitivity, like that of a human hair or that of a soap bubble, to listen to this, the still small voice of a heart. Or the sensitivity of someone like Dario Robleto. Remember his vigil beside the bed of his dying grandmother: it is the same, I think, as the soap bubble or the human hair. It takes a lot of heart to listen attentively to so slight and quiet a force as this, the beating of a heart. Robleto's is as sensitive as a human hair and a soap bubble.

*September 17, 2018.*
    *"I can't go on, you must go on, I'll go on, you must say words. . . . You must go on, I can't go on, I'll go on." (Samuel Beckett,* The Unnamable, *final lines)*

    *As a college teacher, I meet a lot of young people who are rightly disheartened by the cold, steely heart of the world they expect awaits them in our overly managerial, overly managed society. These students are tempted to turn to easily consumed, pretty packages of experience and identity offered as compensation. Jeff Koons's hearts are always available. It's very attractive, I have to admit. But this, too, one might expect, will soon lose its shine. In the absence of more and more such shiny hearts, one might reach the breaking point, the heartbreaking point where one realizes that having lost their shine, these hearts are themselves full of hot air.*
    *In that heartbreaking point, if we let it break, we might, however, find what it feels like to have a heart. That is hard, a hard lesson to learn and an even harder way to learn it. I don't want to do it. I wish I didn't have to. And I hesitate to teach it, I hesitate to let it be taught, but the youth, and any of us, who fear having a heart because it might break need to know that: Yes, it is hard to have a heart. But that need not be cause for despair, nor need it be the cry of despair. Just because it's hard to have a heart, we need not harden ours and steel ourselves. It is hard to have a heart, they break, they are constitutively defective, they are found to be lost, but I also need to have a heart, an open one, maybe even a warm one, to take heart . . .*

*Lexington, VA, August 26–September 17, 2018*

# INTERLUDE

# AFTER THE FACT

*November 5, 2018.*

*It's November. One of the things I am doing as I struggle to come back to my senses is make sense of what I was doing in the weeks before, before the surgery that gave me the possibility of a future.*

The words you read in the preceding pages were written in large part during a few weeks before I had open-heart surgery. The impending event lent a necessity and a significance to everything that was happening around me, the fall of every early autumn leaf meant as much as the fall of Rome. I had to do something, I felt, to attend to the reality happening around and to me, to not miss the facts of my situation, to be awake to what was dawning in, with, and over me. Writing was the answer, this writing, that writing about the heart and what it feels like to have one. You might have sensed the urgency.

I could not always seize the moment every moment; my heart wasn't strong enough for that, and I lost focus, missed the train of thought, watched it pass into the distance of the day and its night, then slept. You might have sensed that, too, in the incompleteness. The time was interrupted by various appointments and decisions, meetings and consultations, but it was by and large free time, and even if I was not always able to seize the days, there were lots, though running out, and they were long, though certain to end. I worked on it as best I could, with some amount of coherence, until I had to stop. I am glad now to have the chance to continue.

Much of what I wrote was new, but there was also much that built on thoughts I had wrestled with in notebooks and journals dating back several years. The encounters with the artworks, for instance, date from the summers of 2015 and 2016. I had been approaching art objects in terms of the heart since early 2015 when, on the basis of my book *Arts of Wonder: Enchanting Secularity*, I was invited to contribute an essay to a collection that would be devoted to seeking spirituality in contemporary art. Although I was fired from that project even before beginning it, because, to paraphrase the curator, *heart* is too far out there even for a project that intends to go out on a limb by engaging spirituality, I nevertheless continued to think about what I had called "art with a heart" and sketched some thoughts around that theme in various notebooks. The notebooks sat unopened for several years until the unavoidable confrontation with my defecting, my broken heart threw me back upon these things of the past. Opening the notebooks again a couple months ago, I found those thoughts. Now, however, they were mine: they were not abstract engagements with ideas about the heart as seat of emotion, nor were they considerations of objects, works of art in historical settings. Thoughts once just entertained now concerned me in a more urgent now. Matters of the heart that I thought belonged to a past that was behind me now clearly lay ahead of me in a future that was coming straight for me.

What could we do in the meantime—between the time of deciding for the surgery we hoped would give a future and that

undecided future? Wait. My future was not one I was making
so much as one whose arrival I could only wait for. Writing, writing those words you just read, I see now, was a practice of that
waiting, keeping open—an open heart? It's not that writing took
action; it's more that with writing the passivity of waiting became
creative, generative. Given my failing heart, it was about all I
could do—not to kill time but to work with it. Surgery, the big
event, was still up ahead of me and after that . . . it, too.

I had to write—and so I did write—and so at last I could
write. It was the way to take up matters of the heart as my own,
an appropriation I had not been called to do previously in the
notebooks and hadn't; the notebooks had lain closed for a long
time. What I wrote during those few weeks of waiting felt less
like what I wanted to say than what I had to say. That's why I
have to read the pages again now to make sense of them. Where
were those words coming from? Did they make sense, and if they
did was it sense I wanted or intended? I was and am often surprised and even scared by what I wrote and am writing, terrified
by some of the thoughts that came and come up, and yet I realize that what I did not intend is nevertheless mine. I have to own
up to it and its strangeness—in writing.

One of the things that strikes me when I read those words now
after the fact and from a calmer time and place, is the shifting
tense and mood in which it is written. I vacillate, waver, am
inconsistent, am, in short, moody. It was hard, having the heart
to write about mine, those days, and I could not remain steady
faced with that uncertainty.

I see now that I write then about the future, surgery and its
aftermath, from two different perspectives or points of view:
sometimes tranquilly from somewhere else than the present

looking at that future, so as to see it as if it were the accomplished past; but also sometimes as if it were an uncertainty experienced in the urgent now. Consider this:

> *But that's hard to do, I am finding, when your heart is at issue. / Having decided on the critical care of my heart, what will be the outcome of this medical intervention? Sure, complication rates are 2 percent or less, but am I one of the 98 percent? Having chosen to take up the burden of my defective heart with this intervention, what sort of life will we be making? What if I feel the same after the intervention? Is that still success? It might work, but it might not. In the case that concerned me, mine, it might not work for me. I could be one of the 2 percent. Having decided to fight, which side will be victorious, I wondered—like the Christian Saint Augustine in his Confessions, where he gives voice to his own anxiety about the heart that he takes up in the act of conversion.*

Here in this example, the tense begins in the present ("that's hard to do, I am finding") and the mood is characterized by the inter-rogative questioning of a saying performed in that present, the present where one is faced with the future and uncertainty ("What will be the outcome . . ." "Am I one of the 98 percent . . ." "It might . . . it might not . . .")—until the final sentences: "In the case *that concerned* me, mine, it might not work . . ." where a past tense creeps in and finally dominates in the final clause: "which side will be victorious, *I wondered.*" That ending is an indicative in which I don't state my uncertainties about the out-come as a present worry but as a past one. Where is that spoken from? It is as if by the end of the passage, I am writing from a future that I have already reached, or from a moment outside the time when the uncertainty is performed, recollecting in tranquil-ity the worried emotion of the past. In short, it as if I am writing about the worry over the uncertain outcome of my struggle from a moment when that outcome has been decided, and decided in my favor, victory! The present has vanished and with it all the urgency and all the worry—in short, all the still outstanding future. This is, I think, the tense and the assertion of a dream, a wish-fulfillment, one that hides its status as a wish, using the indicative mood to hide the fact that it is a wish and obliviate the question it denies in answering. Putting the worry about the future in the past, asking the question from a position in which it has been answered—these obviously settle the anxiety of the present, lift me out of it, and bring a certain steadiness and a steady certainty to my restless heart.

I see something similar when I write, "This is not even to mention the one big, obvious question that shadowed the expectations that made up our days: What if it doesn't work? What if they put me in a coma, cut me open, and can't put me back together again?" Terrifying ideas, thoughts that can only be thought in fear and trembling, worry and anxiety. I say that these thoughts "shadowed the expectations that made up our days." When did I write that? Where was I, when was I, when those thoughts were written? Why the past tense, "shadowed" and "made up our days," when I was at the time living those days before surgery? I could have written that they "make up our days," for they did, they did make that present for us. Yet I surely wished to be somewhere else when writing, somewhen else, beyond the present situation in a time and place when it was all over and done with without ever having had to go through it. In writing, here and throughout, did I slip into a fulfillment of that wish?

Healthy-minded?

The essay vacillates. It's not always so "healthy-minded," perhaps that is its health. In some places, yes, the prose does seem written as "emotion recollected in tranquility," as my friend Jim pointed out. Then the tense appears to be the past written from a moment that belongs to some form of wishful thinking, a moment of achieved future without further future. At other times I write in a present about the undecided future. Then the prose is more worried, the emotion more emotional. For example, the start of the passage previously examined:

> *Having decided on this critical care of my heart, what will be the outcome of this medical intervention? Sure, complication rates are 2 percent or less, but am I one of the 98 percent?*

Or else the passage that runs like this:

> *They will cut out the valve I was born with and stitch in a new one. . . . They will also cut out a segment of my ascending aorta. It has an aneurysm that makes it thin and weak. They will replace it with a tube made of Dacron, a material used in fishing lines, clothing, and firehoses. Without these, I will not live, at least not very much longer.*

Here the declarations are made from a perspective in the present from which the question as to which side the victory lies remains undecided, a perspective that does not see from beyond the urgent now of the world of concerns weighing on me with the future. It is written in a very different mood than the statements that see the worry as if after the fact from a dreamed-of moment beyond the future, a moment in which victory has been decided.

This variation is not the effect of editing or revision. It belonged to the present to which I was attuned by the writing. It came with attentiveness to the present of worry focused on the uncertain outcome of the now, which is also the present that gives ground, ambiguously, to hope and wishful thinking: hopeful anticipation writing in the midst of the anxiety I was writing about as if I had survived and passed through it and was recollecting it tranquilly. The worried present gives ground to hope, but it frequently happens that in giving ground to hope, it yields entirely, collapses under all those hopes, and we live entirely in gleeful optimism, hoped-for and dreamed-of worlds oblivious of the worried realities they are made to address. I am trying now, it seems, to convince myself that some form of wishing is legitimate, some form of hoping comes from eyes wide open not only from denial and despair but from a worried heart taking on critical care for the present.

It is tempting to leap out of the vacillation, oscillation, and unsteady present of having a heart. Augustine did. He doesn't always speak from the place of confession I identified two or three months ago. He doesn't always speak in a heartfelt way, for instance, of his uncertainty as to "on which side victory lies" or his longing for mercy and assistance. Sometimes his wishes are stated dogmatically and no longer appear as wishes. When not confessed, they take form as dogmatic certitudes that have lost their ground in the anxiety and worry out of which wishes come; the ground has given ground and gives way. I can understand that temptation, but I tried to resist it in a writing that remained attentive to the present world of concern and worry, writing from the heart, and so wavered.

A good example of the more dogmatic Augustine is the famous *City of God*, especially the final chapter, in which he speaks knowingly about the happiness of the final end and the conviction that access to it comes to Christians through the strength of their belief. The book is conceived as a theodicy—that is, an attempt to justify the belief that God is in control of history despite the fact of Rome's disastrous fall. (Who could believe after that?) This belief being justified, believers can rest assured that all that happens is good since brought by a divine cause. Which means that the evils that seem to befall believers are only apparent evils, perspective errors that when seen from the correct point of view, the divine point of view, are cleared up and known to belong to God's plan for the good. Helping us see history truly (planned by God) is the task of the book. Almost the entire work is composed as answers to questions a restless heart might ask about the history of life, both individual life and the life of mankind over the course of history: the nature of its end, a depiction of its beginning, the reason for its present misery, the basis for confidence that the promise of its future felicity will be fulfilled, the means to that fulfillment, and so on. Along the way Augustine offers clear answers to metaphysical questions that subtend being historical and the problem of suffering posed by it: the freedom of the will, the need for the baptism of infants, the intercession of saints in salvation, and so on. What you have to do is believe them, the answers and their teachers and He in whose name the teacher teaches. That would be enough to settle the heart's uncertainty as to the outcome of the matters that vex it. This is what the doctrinal and metaphysical discussions in *City of God* do. They let the heart know what it believes so that it can see and have the victory that otherwise in life with its restlessness remains as yet undecided. Such having in advance is what it means to hope, Augustine says, but this believing hope sounds to me like "to expect," a way to be toward the future in which the present uncertainty about the outcome is lifted and replaced with a "not yet," not yet realized or actualized end I know (expect) will turn out.

Reading *City of God*, listening to Augustine speak in it, I feel as if the restless heart has already reached the point where it rests in peace. This achievement is possible because the author of the book views matters from a time beyond history (the end of time, Judgment Day) and a place beyond the world (the New Jerusalem). From the viewpoint of this divine time and place the heart sees without worry how things turn out and for whom they turn this way and for whom they turn that way.

The name I would give to our means of access to that time and place is "Belief." Belief of any kind: belief in what the word of God (prophets, psalms, Revelation, Genesis, and so on) has informed us of, whether directly in revelations or through the church and its doctrine or some combination of both; but also the belief of those who tell you it will all be okay, that the pounding in your head is not a sign that the surgery has failed or, worse, succeeded in bringing threats of stroke. Belief lets us see from the point of view of the one who, outside the thick of things and no longer in the heart of it all, sees from the perspective of the end, when questions have been answered, all the evidence is in, and judgments have been made deciding which side was victorious. Even if I am not there yet, belief lets me see what is seen by the one who is.

Unlike Augustine, I don't think of myself as much of a believer. Where are they speaking from when they tell me it will be all right, that it was a success, that the pounding in my head is not an imminent disaster? Belief might already have its future in the present so that it can write about the future as past, calmly, therefore, *knowing on which side victory lies* and moreover that it lies with me. What is at present lacking in itself (*in se*) is, for the believer, had in hope (*in spe*) that believes, but as nonbelieving, I don't find that this sounds much like the hope I know, at least not like the experience of the miserable condition of hope that I *knew*. I found it difficult to access and impossible to maintain a position from which to see as believers do. I could, however, and did, I see upon reflection, dream of it in writing, but the dream

would last only for a while, and I would wake to present realities, pressing unavoidably on me in the form of missed beats, a
swelling chest, pounding head, or stolen breath. The mood of my
writing vacillates, therefore, like my attention, present or
dreaming—dreaming because present? That vacillation springs
from tending to what it feels like to have a heart.

The weekend before surgery I shared my essay at heartening
thoughts with a few close friends, then shortly after I returned
home to begin recovery there, I shared it with more. That wid-
ening circle included those friends who had reached out from
elsewhere with wishes for my health, requests to hear about it,
or just reminders of their presence, however distant. Their words
from afar touched me quite closely, so closely that I would often
respond by sending these pages to them. One of those friends
was Tria, who lives some seven hundred miles away in Chicago.
I met her twenty years ago when I began working in the office
of the theater where she was a principal performer and instructor. Tria is anything but a colleague. She has not read much in
philosophy or religious studies, the fields in which I count my
expertise, and she is not theoretically informed. Expert of nothing I know anything about, she is not someone I would ever meet
in professional circles. She is a friend.

Tria responded to my response, and we corresponded,
responding back and forth to each other. Shot through with
delays and deferred replies, our communication was anything but
simultaneous, synchronous, or a shared presence in the present
to each other. It was hardly facetime and nothing near a face-to-
face, yet the lag in time and the distance in space, so little appre-
ciated in a technological milieu of instant messaging, ongoing
notifications, and next day delivery, did not impede and maybe
even belonged to what proved a heartfelt exchange.

"The most important and basic thing" in that exchange, as Tria put it, was to say, "I had in fact read and reread your letter." Hearing that mattered more than what she thought about the contents of such letters. Hearing that was more touching than knowing she comprehended or agreed with what was said in those letters. It was the weight of it mattering and the sense of it touching, just the fact of "in fact, I read it," that proved heartening, vital and vitalizing, to me. It might be what is meant when we say something is heartfelt: the heart, where the effect of touch and mattering is felt even and especially across distances of time and space.

It is the same with lovers who say "I love you" without knowing what that means but care only that it is being said to each other. This alone is what matters, when you are my heart, as was the case for Simon and Juliette in a book I read this month, Maylis de Kerangal's beautiful novel *The Heart*: "They used to stay up late, talking into the night while the house was asleep, and maybe they would even whisper I love you, not really knowing what it was they were saying, only that they were saying it to each other, that was what mattered, because Juliette—Juliette was Simon's heart."[1]

From the distance in which our heartfelt friendship transpired, I learned something important about the writing I had undertaken two months ago. Tria wrote this:

The thing about the grace of your writing—
it is its own shiny, wonderful and endearing package.
In some ways it makes you just as criminal as Mr Koons.

Because the true weight of the ragged heart (which I know you are
experiencing and talking about)
means you don't even have a way to mouth this essay.

I was pleased to hear this, but I was also startled and chal-
lenged. What was startling was the observation that, in effect,
the essay was impossible to write truthfully, her implication that
the weight of the ragged heart taken on should be experienced
in an anxiety that, lacking words, can at best only cry. Yet I had
not cried. I had written, she said, with "grace," eloquently and
beautifully, "a shiny, wonderful, and endearing package." Was it
a lie, then, feigned feeling or deceptive appearance?

How does anyone mouth the fears and uncertainties that
come with having a heart, especially when its constitutive defect
is laid bare? How to stick words to incomprehensible experiences without purpose: the advent of my own death or the sense
and reason for my own birth, the inexplicable stealing away of a
child from its mother's arms by a tsunami wave, Hitler, the
freakishness of a two-headed snake, the experience of divine
transcendence? The meaning of my broken heart? It is an old
question; philosophers and especially theologians have wrestled
with it for millennia. I don't think I have much to add, except
maybe myself. Tria would say in subsequent correspondence,
"the fact seems to me that there is no language at the center of
those moments."

Without language, such moments, in fact and to speak truthfully, mean nothing, they are empty, as empty as . . . well, nothing, for in sticking a word to them or figuring them with images
or metaphors or similes that make them like something else, they
mean something (that which they are like or that which they are
said to be in words) and become part of a world made up of such
significant references. Figuring it out might be something I do
when I write or speak and thereby assign language to the facts,
but it is not the facts, not the real fact as it was suffered by me.
On their own and left to themselves, without me and the sense

I make of it, the facts in truth are just themselves, reality just is reality. The truth is, the facts are, heartbreak is heartbreak, without reprieve, relief, or release. All hearts are defective, life is lived with an expiration date, I learned, our open hearts have skeletons inside, the last beat will beat the last and nothing, only nothing, comes of that. "Merciless is the beating heart," Karl Ove Knausgaard writes. "The heart beats, and then it does not. That's it."[2] Those are the facts, the ugly truth. The "ragged heart" that all hearts are at heart is itself nothing more than that.

If I want to face the facts head on, that means seeing them without all the graceful writing and language that makes sense not reality of it. The closer I get to the reality of what it means to have a heart, the less pretty things really become and the more a betrayal of that reality the writing is, especially graceful writing. The reality is this, as Knausgaard says in the first words of his six-volume, 3,600-page *My Struggle*: "For the heart, life is simple: it beats for as long as it can. Then it stops. Sooner or later, one day, this pounding action will cease of its own accord."[3] It's "merciless," as he says, but "that's it." That's just how it is: hearts beat, then they stop. Without why. Too tired to go on but not yet at the end, they stop. The reality that Knausgaard draws near, like the one to which I hoped to attend, is the fact of the constitutively defective heart whose beating stops "of its own accord." He did it for 3,600 pages! Everything else we say about the heart and living with one is in excess of that reality, a fiction, and I have written quite a bit more than that truth. I have written about having a heart, a heart that is at bottom heartbreak, not mercilessly but "gracefully," offering "shiny," "wonderful" language that was, Tria said, quite beautiful. A heartbreaking reality was replaced with a lie, a charming, graceful picture, a fiction, literature.

What are we doing when we struggle to write words that come from the heart where reality is taken on? Can we live without that language? Much of book 6 of Knausgaard's *My Struggle* is a struggle with those questions. Tria's thoughts raised them for me. It didn't hurt that I was reading Knausgaard, too, at the time. Was what I had done in this essay a betrayal of the truth of experience, a lie that had taken the ugly, painful reality of my defective heart and presented in its place beautiful, graceful language that felt meaningful? Was it deceptive, was I tricking readers and myself that way? Was I "just as criminal as Mr Koons" in telling stories or writing fictions about heartbreaking moments, charming others and deceiving myself?

After a delay that was characteristic of our ongoing heart-to-heart, I tried to write back. It wasn't easy; matters of the heart aren't. Because they don't flow easily, there will always be delays in the to and fro of the passing from heart to heart and back again differently. Because the heart is weighty, the exchange that takes it on will be heavy and drag slowly. It is painful to write about much of this; of course, there will be hesitations and delays.

My hesitant response to Tria has been incorporated into what you are reading. I have not been shy about that. I want to show the life in which thoughts arise and play themselves out, offering a reminder that they do arise in the course of our living a life and that they radiate out and shape our being in the world. My own experience has been that thoughts come up, often without my first thinking them and often without my willing or wanting them to come up. Do they come from the heart, then, an open, sensitive heart? We should not hold that unwilled origin or unmanaged course against them and dismiss them, for in dismissing the thoughts that come up from elsewhere and

unexpectedly we miss the opportunity to live thoughtfully—
and may also fail to have a heart.

Writing was one way to expose myself to thoughts that come
from the heart. Friendship was another, the heart-to-heart in
which I don't so much tell my secrets or spill my guts (heart is not
gut) as undergo the thoughts that come up in me from afar. My
friendship with Tria being one case, but there were and are others. An important form our friendship took was our correspondence. Thoughts were shared in letters sent across distance—or
rather, thoughts came up as they were shared in the letters that
sent them across distance. It would be a mistake to imagine I first
thought these thoughts, knew the things I had to say, then gave
them material form in letters. In fact, the thoughts came to me in
letters I shared with friends across the distance they opened in
and for me—a heart-to-heart from which thoughts come.

Tria made me aware that my writing might make "graceful"
something that is "merciless," might make wonderful something
that is just the ugly truth. In treating matters of the heart gracefully, I was not doing justice to them. Justice is "merciless," the
opposite of mercy and grace, as everyone trained in theology
knows. I was conflicted with this realization. Again, was it criminal? It made me think of a passage from the philosopher Friedrich Nietzsche's book *The Gay Science*, and so I turned to the page
where he writes, "As an aesthetic phenomenon existence is still
*bearable* for us" (§107). The remark is made in the course of a
reflection on the rise of science to tribunal of reality, the arbiter
passing judgment on what counts as real. Science stands more
broadly for what Nietzsche calls elsewhere "the will to truth," to
not know the false but also and more fundamentally to not lie,
not even to oneself, to not be deceived or to deceive oneself.

Embedded in this is also the assumption that truth is reached by a knowledge that gets behind or beneath appearances, appearances that are always deceptive covering over a hidden truth. An ethical imperative or teaching about how to live therefore comes along with this scientific attitude to reality, Nietzsche suggests: namely, the imperative to unmask or demystify appearances so as to live lucidly in the truth and its light. When reality is accessed in true knowledge, this ethical teaching says, sticking to the truth, not letting appearances gain the upper hand and mask it, is the good life.

That teaching is realized in a character Nietzsche presents in his great work *Thus Spoke Zarathustra*, the Soothsayer (*der Wahrsager*), literally the one who speaks the truth truly.[4] Fixed on the truth of reality, saying only what he knows and knows is true, the Soothsayer actualizes the ethical teaching implied by the will to truth, but he is also what Nietzsche calls "the proclaimer of the great weariness." Listen to what the speaker of truth is teaching when we first meet him: "All is empty, all is the same, all has been. . . . In vain was all our work." And when he returns at the end of the book: "All is the same, nothing is worth while, the world is without meaning, knowledge strangles." What is is only itself, he says wearily, all is the same; x always and only x, truly nothing, meaning nothing more; the truth is: all is in vain.

In a soothsayer, knowledge of the truth appears in and brings great weariness, despair and melancholy. As Nietzsche puts it in *The Gay Science*, "*Honesty* would lead to nausea and suicide" (§107). If our lives are formed only by true knowledge of the true, if we only give voice to what we know lies behind appearances, if we are soothsayers, we will grow sick and nauseated at having a heart, for "merciless is the beating heart . . . The heart beats and then it does not. That's it." They are all constitutively defective; mine bears an expiration date; it's only a matter of time. Taken as such, in all honesty, that truth is impossible for me to digest. Suicide is an understandable temptation, Nietzsche suggests—understandable to those with a heart that has not been hardened or grown steely or heartless. There is a sign of life, then, a sign of a heart beating faintly, in the experience of that temptation and those who dream of it. But it needs to be said, too: the release sought is not one the actual suicide is there to experience or enjoy, despite what popular books and television shows like *13 Reasons Why* might lead one to believe. Entertaining shows like that make suicide attractive by affording an impossible perspective (a transcendent perspective, a believer's perspective?), an impossible point of view of life after life, where surviving my suicide I benefit from it. The temptation is satanic when presented this way?

Still, it would be heartless of me to deny the temptation of release apparently offered by such an escape when having a heart is heavy as it is. The experience of the temptation to suicide, then, indicates something worth saving, and so the tempting possibility is *not* taken while still experienced as temptation by a still beating heart that feels the truth: "the heart beats and then it does not. That's it." The heart that experiences the temptation still has a pulse. It is the heart worth saving. Suffering the temptation should mean a heartfelt recoil.

One form taken by that heartfelt recoil is art—where despair and melancholy, nausea and the temptation to suicide are resisted. The Soothsayer's knowledge is had, Nietzsche tells us, in a mood that despairs of the ugly truth. Art, by contrast, is a "counterforce against our honesty that helps us avoid such consequences: art as the *good* will to appearance. We do not always keep our eyes from rounding off something and, as it were, finishing the poem; and then it is no longer eternal imperfection that we carry across the river of becoming—then we have the sense of carrying a *goddess*, and we feel proud and childlike as we perform this service." The eternally imperfect because constitutively defective heart, for instance, can be taken up and carried through world and time in artful appearances. With these graceful appearances, Nietzsche says, we are made to feel—and how we feel matters, mood an important consideration, the heart not to be neglected—we are made to feel that our journey through life is "carrying a goddess through a river." This fiction, these creations or works of art, are not alternative facts, they do not deny the truth of what the soothsayer spoke verily, "merciless is the beating heart; . . . it beats for as long as it can. Then it stops." If art is a heartfelt recoil before the temptation to suicide, that recoil should not be understood as averting the gaze or turning around in flight but as something more like a wide-eyed step back, a retreat that keeps sight of the facts and holds onto the ugly truth all the while it creates beautiful work with it. This is how one recoils gracefully, neither spastically in terror nor gleefully in ignorance and blindness.[5] In the graceful work of art, the imperfection of reality, the ugly truth that we admit when we are honest with ourselves, the facts of our congenital defects and constitutively broken hearts—all is taken up as a goddess. In such a work, the ugliness of the truth does not count against life. How you bear it, how you feel while carrying the truth, matters.

This is why Nietzsche says, in *The Gay Science*, that existence is "*bearable*" as an aesthetic phenomenon. "Bearable" stands as a marked departure from an earlier formulation. That earlier formulation, as noted by the translator, Walter Kaufmann, appears in *The Birth of Tragedy* (twice, §§5, 24) and reads, "it is only as an aesthetic phenomenon that existence and the world are eternally justified." In changing "justified" to "*bearable*," the revision no longer asks existence to render reasons that would justify it, as if there were a tribunal other than it before which existence must defend its legitimacy. This means also that the revision avoids presenting aestheticization as a defense of existence, as if a positive judgment about the facts depended upon them being made beautiful by art. In short, the revision moves away from a situation in which existence stands under accusation and one uses art to brighten it up and aesthetics to judge the pretty picture made. In this departure, Nietzsche's revision tries to approach the innocence of existing in a world that is beyond justification because beyond good and evil—in effect, a world before and without me and my judgments, the facts.

The issue, Nietzsche came to realize, is not justification of existence but how we bear reality now, how we bear the facts of existing in a world that is beyond justification because at bottom beyond meaning and meaninglessness, how we are in this chronic condition of being in the world. This is not a scientific or epistemological question but a practical one, a matter of the practice of life today, now. Recognizing the urgency of the concern, Nietzsche speaks of world and existence being "still *bearable*." *Still* because we are in the world and have to bear it today, through a river of time, not an unchanging eternity of heaven. Whether or not and even if, existing is justified for all eternity, I still have to bear it today, in time and the times, which keep recurring, again and again until they don't, asking again and again in each moment if I can *still* bear it, still. This is, I think, a question of your heart.

A response to this practical question is made by art, what I have been calling graceful appearances, which Nietzsche thought could give us "the sense of carrying a *goddess* . . . across the river of becoming" and time. If taking on the burden of existing means "carrying a goddess," who would not rally to the task, who would not feel called upon to awaken from the great weariness—who would not find that a heartening thought? Only the most heart-less of unbelievers, only the most convicted devotees of a truth laid bare in a knowledge that demystifies, or else only those true believers who are, they, too, disheartened by the defects of exist-ing, those true believers who because of its defects can't believe it is a goddess and are incapable of praising it as such . . . that's who: they would not take heart.

Artful presentations do not make the facts of life perfect or more fulfilling. Gracefully presenting heart failure as the truth of having a heart, I can take it up in the way I would take up a goddess, with pride and the innocence of a child, as if my fail-ing life was worship, what Nietzsche calls a service or act of devo-tion. This makes it "still *bearable*." It does not alter the ugly truth, and it does not offer reasons that justify it, but when the ugly truth is presented "gracefully," I am not paralyzed by it, am not given over to despair by it, but can go on, onward, with it—and getting on with it is crucial in the midst of a broken heart. My essay, this book, is, in its style and form, "my struggle" to take up the ugly truth of having a heart in ways that make us (just me?) feel as if we are carrying a goddess when we pick it up and bear it across, through, into the river of time that still rushes on.

*Lexington, VA, November 5–22, Thanksgiving Day, 2018*

# I

# BOOK OF MY HEART

*December 2018.*

*Hearing of my struggle to write about what it feels like to have a heart, a friend who is editor at an important university press sent me, just before my surgery, a book he had seen to publication. It was called* The Book of the Heart, *written by Eric Jager, a medievalist. My friend called my attention to several images it contained of heart-shaped songbooks, prayer books, and books of hours; they were part of the devotional life of the religious and frequently dedicated to conversion or a change of heart. He told me further that this is where he learned that the figure of speech "turning over a new leaf" comes from these objects. He said he looked forward to hearing from me after I opened a new chapter of my own.*

*The title alone was irresistible:* The Book of the Heart. *Could that be what I am writing? Yes and no, for the book I am writing does include a lot about the heart, but it is also the heart I call mine. It is not only "the book of the heart" but also "the book of my heart." What difference does it make? What difference does it make when the heart becomes my heart, something you too can say? Mine has been stopped, torn open, and cut up in the process of changing it, opening its next new chapter.*

# 1

# THE HEART I CALL MINE

Theology tells about the book of the heart. It is where the story of your life is written. All that you say and do, all that you think and feel, is recorded there in your heart. Many early and medieval Christians connected the word for heart (*cor*) etymologically with the word for record (*re-cordor*), making it easy to depict the heart as a record, a book recording who I am and what I did, my very self. Eric Jager writes,

> a key Western metaphor of selfhood . . . portrayed the individual's life as a narrative that is "written" in the "books" of both personal memory and divine omniscience. . . . Memory or "conscience" as an interior "writing" came together in early Christian theology, which evoked for the first time a book of the heart containing a moral record of the life of the unique individual. This inner book could be read (and even revised) in pursuit of self-understanding, but it remained under divine purview, and it would be "opened" for a final and very public reading at the Last Judgment.[1]

Later in his study Jager observes that whereas early Christianity held that the record recorded in the book of the heart was of the moral life, medieval thinking held that the book also contained a record of the affective life, the emotions, feelings, thoughts and passions that constitute who we are. Either way, regardless of its plot or central conflict, the book of the heart is a cumulative record containing the story of my life, the memory that makes me who I am. That story, in its theological telling, has an end, not the end of my life on earth in worldly time but the apocalyptic eschaton or end of world and time. This end, theology conceives not as curtain drop but as arrival at or else arrival of the final destination—*telos* more than *finis*.

The end of the story is also known as Judgment Day or the Last Judgment. At that time, the book of the heart is put in the hands of God to be weighed, finally, once and for all eternity, so that a judgment can be issued deciding its final final resting place. The earliest depictions of this scene show the book of the heart being taken from each of us, opened, and read publicly by angels so that God can hear the testimony recorded in it. By the late Middle Ages and early modern period, however, individuals themselves put their book on scales held in God's hands to be weighed and judged. The book of the heart is in our hands, it seems, at least in the days before the Last Judgment. It is written by us, by our thoughts and deeds, feelings and desires. These make us who we are, and who we are is recorded in and *as* the book of the heart.

But even if the book of the heart is in our hands, the medieval theologians tell me, we are not always in full knowledge, and sometimes not even aware at all, of what we are writing. Much of its writing happens in secret and that secret is kept even from myself. When I take my heart into consideration, then, I don't know entirely what I am doing or who I might be. God, however, sees it differently because from another point of view, one from which he can know what is in my heart. This is noted expressly by Hraban Maur, a monk, later the abbot of Fulda then archbishop of Mainz, someone that neither I nor anyone I know had ever heard of but who is cited by Jager. Hraban spoke of a book "hidden in our heart, containing written records of our deeds and marked, so to speak, with the reproofs of conscience, and still known to no one but God. But these books of our soul or tablets of our heart shall be opened before the throne." What is remarkable about the story recorded in Hraban's heart is that though it is his, the story of who he is, even a story of which he is more or less the author, he does not know all that is written in it. My heart has secrets, he says. Intriguingly, Hraban names "God" the keeper of secrets, the secrets of my heart, my most intimate intimacy unknown to me.

Your heart keeps secrets, then, even from yourself—at least until Judgment Day, when, Hraban says, the book of the heart is "opened before the throne." The secrets of the heart are not ultimate mysteries, at least not for this theology: you don't take them just to the grave with you but *beyond* the grave to Judgment Day when the veils keeping the secrets secret will be lifted by their divine keeper. St. Ambrose says as much: "That which has always been apparent to the Lord will be clearly revealed on the Day of Judgment, when the secrets of the heart, which were thought to be hidden, will be called to account." Your heart might keep secrets, from you, too, but not for all eternity, only for all time, and time and the days will come to an end, the believers believe. There will be an apocalypse, they say, literally, *apokalupsis*, which means according to the Greek, *apokalupsis* from *apo–*, "away from or remove," and *kaluptein*, "to cover or veil." At the end, there will be an end of veilings, no more secrets, a final day when the secrets of the heart will be revealed, finally, once and for all, subject to judgment, eternal, eternally definitive judgment, deciding and assigning a final resting place.

For this theological vision, the ragged heart with all its secrets and hidden flaws, all the defects and holes that make it hard to bear, is a chronic condition, lasting only as long as there is world and time—that is, only as long as the *saeculum* endures. It is a secular condition, indeed it is the condition known as secularity, but, the medieval story goes on to tell, there will not always be world and time. From this perspective, a chronic condition is good news, a blessed prognosis. It's not forever, that is eternal. You will give up the book of your heart, hand it over finally, and it will no longer be in your hands. Then and there you will set down, lay to rest, the burden of your heart and no longer need carry it. There is a place to rest, a resting place where you can put it.

The medieval version goes on to say that before the end of the days that end, the book of the heart is in our hands. We try our best to write a good one, to tell a better story, to be more conscientious about what gets written on it. After all, *really* after all, we will hand it over for a final decision, a definitive and decisive decision, by the critic of all critics at the final Last Judgment. This lends some urgency to the now in which the book of the heart is written. That sense of urgency is increased when it is believed, as many medieval theologians hold, that the end of the time we have for writing our book comes before it is over. The end of world and time comes when it will, before the end, at a moment decided by God who is outside the times. Jesus will come when He comes. This puts the medieval heart in an unsettled, restless position, for, when the angels and devils "are gathering up the record books of the heart to bring to the divine tribunal as evidence," the medieval Everyman is likely to "reply that his book is not ready," the book of his heart incomplete.

Even if the book of the heart is not ready to be offered when the angels come for it, there is much that can be done to improve it in the meantime. We can write a better book of the heart by participation in the sacramental system, including confession, and also of course by managing our moral lives in accordance with divine law. These offer reliable guides for making the book of my heart conform to the standards of what the Ultimate Critic will judge a good book. They are ways to take our heart into our own hands in the days before the end of world and days, so that we can approach that end with more confidence and security regarding the quality of the heart we will offer.

Jager's account of later medieval piety makes it particularly evident how the religious life was a way to write a better book of your heart. Much of the devotional literature of this later period, he says, revolves around the Cross and Passion of Christ. It frequently describes the believer's heart as site for "a 'transcription' of the sacred wounds to an inward, individual 'copy' of the Passion. As such, the book of the heart embodies an *imitatio Christi* that was no longer limited to a saintly elite but that everyone could aspire to." The heart is nothing but what is recorded on it, purely passionate in other words, a suffering of passion where the believer feels as his own the passion of another, in the ideal case the Passion, the passion of a specific, exemplary other, Christ. The perfect book of the heart would be such a copy. A host of devotional practices were organized around the intention of seeing that what gets written on the heart makes it a book that is ideal, the best, Christlike in suffering its passion. "Prayer accompanied by sacred signs or gestures," Jager notes, "could transcribe Christ's wounds to the individual's heart," writing a book in which "sacred scenes of the Passion [become] devotional passages written on the heart." "Write . . ." was a frequent invocation opening such prayers, beseeching Christ Himself to write the book of my heart with his wounds. If one wants to have the book of one's heart be as accurate a copy as possible, the surest way to success is to have it written by the original exemplar.

Jager's *Book of the Heart* thereby plots a trajectory where the practices of writing the book of my heart become ways to be more in control of what is written in it, more knowledgeable about our writing of it, more deliberate in its construction. As there is less and less secreted away in my heart, I am more and more empowered to know where I stand now, to predict where I will land in the future, and to take steps to achieve a more desirable outcome. I can write a better book of the heart when I know more about what is in it and how it gets there. Hraban Maur seems a thing of the distant past. We have made progress. The trajectory Jager plots is thereby one in which worry about the book of the heart diminishes as control over its writing increases.

This is not the book I am writing. The book of my heart is more like Hraban's in that it is shot through with secrets, but unlike his it is without his expectation of an end. I am not convinced mine has a plot that goes as far as eternity. He would call me miserable, inhabitant of the wretched condition of chronic secularity. No end to the endings. Veils forever over the veilings.

When I look at what is written on *my* heart these days, I see a record that is missing what is arguably the most important moment of my recent life, the change that opened the new chapter my friend had wished for me. That missing moment, my change of heart, is what I am now writing after. How did I get to the point where I can write this book and tell the story of my heart?

I don't really know what happened to me that day, September 18, 2018, when they stopped my heart, cut it open, and changed it in ways that would alter my life and the possibilities that are its future. When I look into the book of my heart, self-understanding comes up short, self-possession is undone, precisely at what could be taken as a decisive turning point in the narrative that is recorded there. Though it may prove to be one of the most decisive events in the story of my life, I cannot tell you about my change of heart. It remains a mystery. Beyond sedated, I was not there when it happened to me. Comatose, I was not present to make any experience of what they were doing to me. It does not belong to my memory, therefore. Likewise, it has no place in my expectations. Even though my days to come will be running through possibilities granted by this life-changing change of heart, it is not an experience I ever expect to remember. Source of what might come, it nevertheless remains a missing page in the understandably ragged book of my heart. It is recorded in my heart as a mystery, buried there, secreted away as in a crypt. My heart, now a crypt!

That does not give me a lot of confidence in the heart I might present at Judgment Day. Have I lived up to my potential? Have I done all that I can? Writing the book of my heart I cannot identify with somebody like Jean-Jacques Rousseau, who professed being ready for Judgment Day to come at any time. Rousseau wrote boldly on the opening page of his autobiographical book, *Confessions*: "Let the trumpet of the last judgment sound when it will. I shall come, this book in hand, to present myself to the sovereign judge. I'll say loudly: here is what I did, what I thought, what I was."[2] Those *Confessions* were what traditionally would be called the book of his heart, but he calls it here just his book. He is right to do so, for though intended to be from the heart, the confidence and assertiveness, the self-possessed self-assertion, belie its belonging to a genre such as "the book of my heart."

Mine is ragged, pages missing or hard to read, obscure. His is not. Rousseau had confidence that on Judgment Day he could present a full account of himself in the heart, the book rather, that he proffered to the divine balance. I don't. He was certain that his memories were certain, that he therefore knows who he is and who he was, and his certainty gives him confidence in walking forward to the end. I don't, and I expect there are a lot of people like me who listening to their heart find they move in mysterious ways toward unknown ends with origins that remain secreted away. Rousseau was confident that even if the end came now, he was ready for it and for Judgment Day, his book complete and already done. I don't. I identify more with the medieval Everyman, who wants more time: twelve years is what he asks for in the medieval morality play that bears his name. That seems human. I can understand it. I certainly don't feel the book I am writing is ready, and I am not ready for it to be done. I would like to delay and defer, keep the end of endings at bay, hold it off and postpone it, by writing, writing more in the book of my heart. Everyman's request for more time to write the book of his heart is understandable, even modest: twelve years seems a small ask.

I am not ready for the end of days, not now. The book of my heart is still being written.

If I am trying to write a book of the heart that is my heart, something you too can say, one of the things it surely means is that it can be cut up and torn open. I let the experts do that to mine as part of its repair. The heart the surgeon discovered beneath his rib spreader is, obviously, an object very different from the precious, sensitive thing we might carry through our days like a goddess. To write the book of my heart, I need to know more about that heart and the tradition to which it belongs.

To that end, I have been reading a lot, a lot of books and articles about the heart and heart surgery, texts that are canonical in the tradition to which we committed ourselves when we decided for aortic valve replacement surgery. I put myself in the hands of the surgeons who minister that tradition, after all. I feel obliged to read its book of the heart, to read from its canon and learn about its founding fathers. That is how one makes one's own a history in which one finds oneself, and I now find myself thrown into a history of the heart to which all that belonged. Though inexpert, I read the expert journals. Though not intending a career in medicine, I read some textbooks, the ones that teach students how to minister medicine to and perform surgery on the heart. I also read some popular accounts written by medical experts who are particularly gifted storytellers.

The reading has proved very strange. The articles and journals have titles with which I am unfamiliar: *The Thoracic and Cardiovascular Surgeon*; "Foreign Bodies in and in Relation to the Thoracic Blood Vessels and Heart: Techniques for Approaching and Removing Foreign Bodies from the Chambers of the Heart." Trained in philosophy and religious studies, I am more accustomed to reading material with titles like *Being and Time*, *Confessions*, "The Question Concerning Technology," *Lectures on the Philosophy of History*, *Discourse on the Method*, or *The Gay Science*. Writing the book of my heart has become an adventure of undoing, leading me out of what might be called my "comfort zone." Trying to learn what happened to me, I am becoming less me. The effort at self-understanding is undoing the self I thought I knew. It makes me uncomfortable.

To tell the truth, I often wish to be doing something more exciting, more deeply meaningful, more exhilarating than reading dry accounts of the mechanics of a heart or the technical details of procedures like hooking up a cardiopulmonary bypass machine and suturing a prosthetic valve. It is hard for me to imagine sharing the devotion of the surgeons and experts who did and do this professionally, but I owe my future to them and respect their dedication.

What have I, an amateur, learned about the heart and the tradition to which aortic valve replacement surgery belongs? Quite a bit, actually, but along with all the information I acquired, a particular mood has settled over me, an atmosphere that colored all the knowledge gained. I was frustrated and disappointed to learn that the heart was just a machine and the operation a now technical procedure, nothing special really. My future, I came to understand, depended on the disenchantment of the heart. That itself was dispiriting. Far from being a site of precious, sensitive reflection, occasion for deeply moving words, my heart functions, or doesn't, like all the other hearts in ways the experts understand very well. It even recovers, I am finding out, according to a schedule they can predict with great accuracy and therefore manage. No secrets there. The book of *my* heart was starting to look like a book of *the* heart. Realizing this was disappointing and disheartening.

I once told a friend that this book was " 'my struggle' to take up the ugly truth of having a heart in ways that make us (just me?) feel as if we are carrying a goddess when we pick it up and bear it across, through, into the river of time that still rushes on." I am finding that's tough to do when having my heart means being part of the history of the disenchantment of the heart.

The surgery that gave me a future is a form of what is known commonly as open-heart surgery. Mine was an aortic valve replacement (AVR). Coronary bypass surgery is another form of open-heart surgery. What distinguishes open-heart surgery from other forms of heart surgery is that the heart is stopped and the protective sac around it cut open so that it is laid bare and its insides can be seen and manipulated. "Direct visualization" of the heart and having it "under direct vision" are phrases often used by the surgeons describing it. To replace my aortic valve, surgeons needed to expose the inside of the heart by transecting the aorta at the point where it connects to the heart in order to remove and replace the leaky valve.

Open-heart surgery is described in many of the books I read and on the websites of the cardiac surgery programs at institutions such as the Cleveland Clinic, the Mayo Clinic, Columbia University Medical Center, the Texas Heart Institute, and others. There are also many, many videos posted on the Internet documenting actual procedures. I have not watched any, but I have looked at lots of photographs, two of which are here.

Whether one is having a valve replaced or an artery bypassed, the procedure is more or less the same up until the point just after the heart is laid bare. It begins with the anaesthetization of the patient, putting her in a comatose state in which she does not respond to or even feel painful stimuli and is also unable to maintain the muscular effort for autonomy, including the muscular

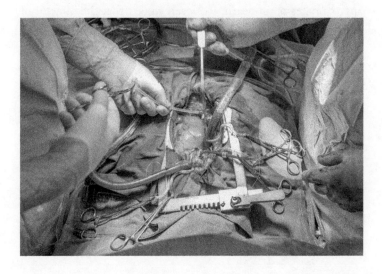

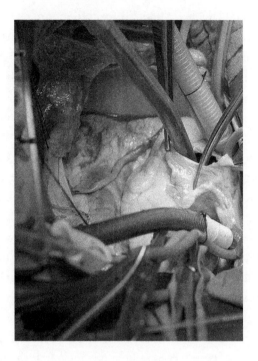

effort needed to maintain respiratory function. This state thereby approximates brain death, so closely in fact that the director of the Heart Failure Program at Long Island Jewish Medical Center, Sandeep Jauhar, describes the beginning of the first open-heart surgery he witnessed by saying, "the patient was anesthetized and intubated, looking like just another cadaver."[3]

Once anesthetic has rendered the patient dead to the world, surgeons cut through the skin of the chest to expose the breastbone. Then, taking up what Jauhar calls a "buzz saw that looks like an ironing press," a surgeon cuts a length of the sternum and with a retractor, a sort of reverse clamp, forcibly separates the two sides of the bone so as to expose the organs previously protected by its cover. What had been secure, hidden away under cover of the ribcage, is unsecured and laid bare.

Seeing the discovered organs clearly now, the surgeon can manipulate the heart. She begins by grabbing with a forceps and taking a knife to the pericardium, the sac surrounding the cardiac muscle. When the pericardium has been cut open, the surgeon can operate directly on the heart laid bare. Catheters are sewn into the right atrium and the aorta, which are then attached to the heart-lung machine that, Jauhar says, "is going to keep our patient alive."

And our patient needs to be *kept* alive because her heart won't be able to do the job anymore: it will be stopped during surgery by what sounds like a deliberately chosen then induced heart attack. Indeed, "Elective Cardiac Arrest" is the title of a 1955 paper by D. G. Melrose et. al. that holds an important place in the canon of open-heart surgery.[4] It describes the first experimental study in stopping the beat of a heart by using potassium-based infusions of blood. Why stop the heart? Somewhat counterintuitively, cardiac arrest is a form of what the experts call "myocardial protection." That is, it is a way to protect the tissue of the heart muscle from damage caused by oxygen starvation during the extended period when the heart is cut off from the body and the blood circulating through it. Surviving on built up stores, a heart that has chosen to be dead for a while uses far less oxygen than one that has to maintain the cellular activity needed to beat.

Over the history of cardiac surgery, various forms of myocardial protection have been used. The first was hypothermia. Cold tissues, like a hibernating animal, require far less oxygen than warm, active ones. Stopping short of a chemical induced execution, hypothermia seems more benign but is ultimately less effective than potassium to stop the heart entirely—assuming one knows how to use potassium correctly. Learning that took some time, some trial and error, and some death. Melrose's use of potassium initially met with many failures and consequent skepticism, therefore. It was discontinued until the 1970s when successful research studies renewed discussion about its use. Further studies and subsequent debate indicated that the problem concerned less the use of cardiac arrest than the specific chemical and dosage that induced it. Today most surgeons use some form of chemical induced cardiac arrest, frequently in conjunction with another option.[5]

Reading these studies and textbooks, I am growing more horrified at what I did with my heart. The surgeon held it in his hands. I had opened my heart and put it in the hands of others who arrested its motions and then restarted them.

Isn't that always the case, though? Doesn't my heart beat out of my control, my most intimately intimate something that moves without me, something that moves me without my first wanting it? I could stop it, if I wanted to, I could take matters into my own hands, make it submit to my command to stop, but only once, once and for all, I could never start it again. The fact that I could stop it only once and for all is a telling sign that it is not available to my mastering it, for the act that exercises mastery leaves me unable to start anything, unable therefore to make use of what I have mastered by starting it so as to turn it into the beginning of something. To let it go on and live, that is being somewhat out of control.

It was fortunate, then, that I did not have to take matters of my heart into my own hands but could put it in the expert hands of others, surgeons who can stop it *and* start it again. I say the surgeons, but it was really a whole world of others: surgeons, nurses, perfusionists, anesthesiologists, not to mention the insurance companies, biotech companies, and, never forget, government using our tax dollars to incentivize and subsidize so much research and expertise; all these had a hold on my heart. But most immediately, to be sure, it was the surgeons. With my heart in their hands, they could do to me and therefore for me what I could not do for myself: stop my heart without that being once and for all, so as to give it back to me, changed.

For a long time, I thought the image of our hearts being in the hands of another to be theological. I imagined that it was the believers, the religious, who imagined there was an other who held our hearts and that this other was the divine other, God. As for the significance of such an image, I thought of it two ways: one, finding your heart in God's hands was the religious act of self-surrender, or else, two, thinking about it more metaphysically, I would interpret it as an image of divine control of the world and our lives, perhaps providence and predestination. When I looked for actual examples of such images, however, I found few to none, and when I read Jager's book, *The Book of the Heart*, I was disabused of my misconception. The vast majority of theological images show that our heart is in our own hands.[6] When it is pictured in God's hands, most commonly in medieval images, it is after world and time have ended, Judgment Day. In the days before Judgment Day, Jager showed me, our heart is in our hands to make ready for being given to God who will weigh it finally and decisively on that final day.

Reformation Protestantism takes up but modifies the picture of the hands that hold our heart. That modification is exemplified by John Calvin's personal emblem, one he used to seal his letters. It shows a heart held in a human hand. Later versions modify the image and include reference to Calvin's motto: *cor meum tibi offero Domine, prompte et sincere* (I offer my heart to you, Lord, readily and sincerely). Three iterations were particularly striking to me, the first from 1545, the second from 1547, and the third, posthumously, from 1566.

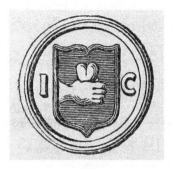
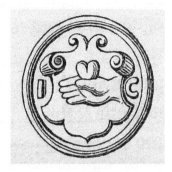

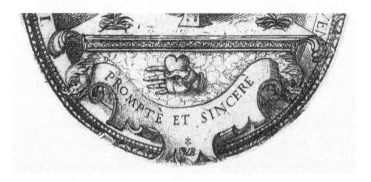

Calvin's emblem with its motto depicts as daily what the medieval images depict as coming only on that one great endless Day that ends the days: namely, the offering of our heart to God. What I see in Calvin's picture is that now, in the present of this world, we take matters of the heart into our hands by giving it over, each day every day, to God. We take up our heart in order to offer it, and we do this daily. Every moment is lived in relation to an end beyond world and time, an end that Calvin knows will come even if he knows not when. Indeed, more than just knowing it will come, he feels it is coming, could come at any moment and therefore offers his heart to God daily, as if every day were the end of days.

The image does not show the decisive moment, the heart being weighed in the balances, only the offering, not its reception, welcome or otherwise, and not the judgment, whether it passes or fails, nor the consequences of either case. Writing the book of *my* heart, I am made restless by such an image. The suspense is worrisome. I worry even now, and I worried even more in August and September as I anticipated handing my heart over to the hands of others. But in none of my reading of Calvin do I sense that he worried. He appears to have had the certainty of knowing that the heart he handed over would be taken up by God, not dropped. He expected that. The very fact that he offered it, he suggests, was a sign that he had already been chosen to have his received and moreover judged favorably. Otherwise, without having been chosen as one of God's elect to receive the gracious gift of Christ that justified him before divine judgment, without being Christian, in other words, he wouldn't even offer it.

In the matter of Calvin's heart, victory has already been decided, then. While judgment has not yet been exercised, the decision has already been made. While the end has not yet arrived, the outcome can be expected. What is more, judgment and outcome can be expected to be positive, a favorable end to the chronic condition of bearing the heart on a daily basis. For Calvin, then, offering his heart, handing it over to the hands of God, is not a matter of putting it at stake in the tilting scales of the balance that weighs it; it is, rather, a matter of glorifying and giving thanks, thanks for the promise that the tilting will stop and that matters settle favorably. Though Calvin still inhabits our chronic condition, his days have already come to an end. The end of time that the medievals (and I) fear lays up ahead was put behind him by Calvin's certainty that judgments had already been made and outcomes already known. When he offers his heart to God in glorification and thanks for His merciful action, Calvin signals to himself and others that his end has already turned out well. That is why he can do it promptly and sincerely, eagerly and with joyful happiness.

The matter of handing over *my* heart was not that convenient nor was it a joy. Like Calvin, I did take my heart into my own hands in order to hand it over, but I did not have his certainty when I gave it somewhat faithlessly and hesitantly, fearfully and with grief, to the hands of mortals who would hold it long enough to repair it. I was putting it in the hands of another before the end of time—at least I hoped it wasn't the end of time. I was giving it over to the hands of others so that I could have more days, not so that I could survive the end of days. I was not offering it to an other beyond world and time so that it could rest safe from the travail of the days and their tribulations. I wanted more days, with all their tribulations, and was somewhat reluctantly and timidly putting my heart in the hands of others who I anxiously hoped would make that possible. I did not know what to expect.

In fact, the others in whose hands I was putting my heart were not just others; they were strangers. I didn't know them at all. I had done my homework, of course, and researched the qualifications of my surgeon and his team. I learned where he received his degrees, roughly how many surgeries he had done, where else he had practiced and so on, but the truth is I don't know anything about him, who he is, what kind of man he is. We talked just once before I let him open me up. He was and remains a stranger—a stranger who held my heart in his hands. When Calvin handed his heart over to the hands of God, he did it knowing full well, he believed, to whom he was giving it over. He did it with certain knowledge—certain knowledge that it was God, identified in Scriptures as Lord, Father, Savior, Creator, to whom he gave his heart. He even had God's Son mediate the relationship and His Spirit seal it so that it was all the more certain than humanly possible. About the only thing I knew for nearly certain about the stranger to whom I was entrusting my heart was that he was *not* God.

When then do we find our heart in the hands of another? When is it that we come to say, "my heart *is* in your hands?" It is a secular statement uttered by one bearing the chronic condition of having a heart. "My heart *is* in your hands" is said when the "you" is a worldly human other. The theologically disposed (the medievals I read about in Jager) take their heart into their own hands, give it only to God and only at the end of time or beyond time, the latter perhaps being indicated by Calvin. In that sense, there never is a time or a day when they say, "my heart *is* in your hands." Not even Calvin, it seems, finds his heart in the hands of another, at least not in a present tense of time as we know it.

Can secularization, then, be understood in terms of a change in who holds our hearts and when we hand them over? A hypothesis: I inhabit the secular condition resolutely and affirmatively when I give my heart to another, find it in the hands of strangers even, in the days before the end of the world and time and therefore without the possibility of a final judgment knowing with certainty once and for all how it will turn out. I am in the world, this *saeculum*, with others, strangers, who hold my heart in their hands.

The prelude to having your heart entirely in the hands of these strangers is attaching the heart-lung machine. Once attached and running, the machine will circulate blood through the body by means of an artificial pump. It will also oxygenate that blood by means of a system of screens, filters, and drips that resembles a still. Blood drains from the body through a cannula inserted into the right atrium, not flowing into the right ventricle where it would get pumped to the lungs. It gathers instead in an extracorporeal reservoir where it is held, ready and on call to be distributed to the body at rates and volumes set by the perfusionist who knows how to manage flows. Under her control, the blood returns to the fleshy body through a system that oxygenates it before it reenters a cannula that had been inserted into the ascending aorta. It then flows through the circulatory system that distributes blood to bodily organs and tissues, driven on by pumping mechanisms located extracorporeally. A portion of the blood that leaves the reservoir and is oxygenated will be diverted through a separate line that both chills it and infuses it with cardioplegic chemicals. Blood pumped through this system returns directly to the heart as arrest-inducing freeze. It enters the heart below the aortic clamp and below the arterial cannula so that it does not mix with the blood being pumped through the rest of the body.[7]

Attaching the life-sustaining machine brings the risk of death. Though the procedure now appears in textbook sections called "Intraoperative Care," when it was first used intraoperatively, it wrought mostly destruction. Seventeen of the eighteen patients on whom early versions were used from 1951 to 1953 died. Even today it is not without its risks, the most significant being a stroke brought on by microemboli dislodged by the pressure of the pumping mechanism running to the brain. Jets and turbulence, pressure gradients and flows, need careful attention. A "sandblast effect" can damage arterial walls or dislodge atheroemboli in seemingly healthy bodies. Aortic dissection can also result as the jet pressing out from the arterial cannula tears the aorta. These risks are managed by preoperative testing and scans that detect high-risk factors like preexisting aortic aneurysms and significant but asymptomatic arterial blockages. Today's heart-lung machine has also been improved—it uses lower pressures than were thought feasible and dual stream catheters to minimize the sandblast effect. The operative complication rate of the heart-lung machine is now less than 1 percent.

Describing the moment when the machine is attached, Jauhar writes, "incredibly the heart began to shrink as blood, life's fluid, was diverted into the plastic-and-metal apparatus. The heart nevertheless continued to beat, though weakly and more slowly." Like any organ or muscle, the heart needs life-sustaining blood to feed it with oxygen in order to work; it loses the strength to contract and therefore pump blood when deprived. The difference between the heart and other organs or muscles is that the heart feeds blood to itself; this is what the coronary arteries do. But, in the preparation for open-heart surgery, not only has a catheter stopped venous blood from flowing into and filling the chambers of the heart (the catheter in the right atrium), but the catheter at the reentry point has also bypassed the heart muscle. As the flow of blood to and from the heart is gradually diverted, the heart slows and shrinks, beating less rapidly and less forcefully. Jauhar observes the approaching cardiac arrest. "Much of my life I'd lived with the fear that the heart could stop at any moment and one's life would be extinguished. And here it was, shrinking like a balloon with a small leak."

When cardiac function is taken over by the machine, the final step can be taken: isolating the heart and stopping its beat. A surgeon uses a metal clamp to compress the aorta, "cutting off blood flow from the heart, thus isolating it. Then he injects ice-cold potassium solution into the main cardiac vein, a dilute form of the same chemical used to stop the heart in executions, and sure enough the patient's EKG quickly flatlines." The potassium solution, a cardioplegia, works by compromising the chemical mechanism that transmits signals across the heart muscle and causes the chambers to contract in an organized rhythm. When this mechanism is disrupted by the potassium solution, the heart quivers chaotically for a brief span of time before it ceases altogether. The surgeon then cools it by pouring iced saline solution over it. The heart has stopped, ceased to beat, frozen in its tracks—as "in executions," Jauhar reminds me.

Throughout the remainder of the operation on the heart, it will stay this way, isolated from the rest of the body and at rest. Its isolation allows a separate perfusion system within the cardiopulmonary bypass machine to deliver cardioplegic solution directly to it without that solution entering the blood that is being circulated through the rest of the body. Most surgeons today favor an intermittent blood-based, hypothermic infusion: the cold temperature of the solution lowers the heart's metabolic demand for oxygen, extending the period during which it can be held in an arrested state, while the blood-based delivery "provides an oxygenated environment and a method for intermittent reoxygenation of the heart."[8] This protects the heart muscle from cellular necrosis induced by oxygen starvation during its arrest while allowing a bloodless field of operation.

Now everything is ready. The surgical field has been prepared. An object is available for expert manipulation, isolated and at rest. *My* heart has become just another heart, *the* heart, in the course of preparing me for the surgery that would give me a future, my future.

The book of my heart depends on this. I could not be writing it otherwise.

If I ever hand over the book of my heart, the event I am describing will likely hold a critical place, the turning point in the story recorded there—or at least *a* turning point, the turning over of a new leaf or the next chapter in my book, as a friend reminded me. Some might even go farther and call it a moment of rebirth, a new beginning, literally, a change of heart. I am generally skeptical of claims to experiences of being born-again, but these days I am playing with the idea. Writing this book might be a way of trying to remain faithful to a change of heart.

Why am I telling this story anyway, writing the book of my heart? Is it to fulfill the autobiographical promise: take possession of yourself in knowing your story; achieve some sort of self-possession or authenticity, maybe even empowerment, in telling the story of your life? Maybe it is to realize some state of self-satisfaction, like the wise man who happily gathers himself together in the present by recollecting his past in a story where the tumultuous events of the past turn out to have been for the good of the present? Those might be good reasons to write the book of the heart at the end of the history Jager describes, but writing the book of my heart has not validated them.

One of the most decisive moments in my book, heart surgery, is a mystery to me, opaque, not just dark but darker than dark. "Beyond sedated, I was not there when it happened to me," I once wrote in a diary. "Comatose, I was not present to make the experience of what they were doing to me." Another darkness besides the darkness that yields to the light of reflection lies at the heart of who I have and will become as faithful heir to that change of heart. Writing the book of my heart, I take on, faithfully?, this mystery—at the heart of who I am.

Heart surgery holds in this way a place like two other events, events without which the story of my life is incomplete: birth and death. While they belong to any and every life story, these two events cannot be narrated in an authentic autobiography. They are not parts of a story I can tell on my own about myself—at least not without consequences that shake the very project of making myself my own. Consider the declarations "I died" and

"I was born," statements that would have to be said if I were to complete the book.

I cannot speak the truth when I say, "I died." Nobody knows the time and place of their death, for it is given to me to know only after I cease to be a knower. Saying "I died," then, requires standing outside my being, becoming an other, in a position possible as what I would call a fiction, be that fiction the fiction of a life after death, the fiction of a self outside its being, or a fiction of the literary imagination. The book of my heart can be completed thanks to a fiction.

Matters become especially interesting to me at the other end of the story of my life: its beginning, birth. I cannot say "I was born on such and such a date in such and such a place" and retain my authenticity. That sentence can be spoken truthfully only by referring to, citing, others—parents, doctors, and nurses, but also legal documents and forms—from whom I heard the truth: "*You* were born on such and such a date." They remember it. I do not. Not being there before it, I was not there to be the one who experienced it and therefore do not have it available in memory for the narration of my life story. My memory of it is theirs. To speak truthfully of my birth, I must cite truths heard from those others who *were* there, when I was not, already expecting me. My birth belongs to their expectations, not mine. It is their expectations that pass into recollections of my birth. I was not there before birth to expect it. It surprised me.

Telling the story of my birth, then, I find myself in the words of others who tell me what I tell myself as my origin. Hearing them say "*You* were born" is the condition of my saying "*I* was born." My story begins with theirs, in which "I" am "You," a second person. My recollection of my birth is theirs. I must become other than I am, become the "You" I hear them say, second person, to tell the story of myself, first person.

If birth does not belong to the expectations of what I am, there is no sense to the declaration, "I will be born." Who is speaking that? And yet I am born, beyond my expectation of the future—miraculously. The I whose story begins with that birth, then, is not the same being as the original I, if "I will be born" can never be said meaningfully. The I who is born is not the same myself, in other words.[9] To begin with, I am an other. My struggle to get close to my origins, to remain faithful to the event that begins my life, to write this book, makes a new beginning of me as I become other than who I am now in the present by telling the story of myself down to its birth.

Could all this be a way to understand my change of heart as a new beginning, a rebirth, a New Being, a new being me? Some did tell me before heart surgery that having never had a heart that functioned optimally, I might not recognize myself when they changed mine. It sounded like religious promises of being born again. I was skeptical and not even sure I wanted to be born again so much as to be who I was then. I wanted to save myself. I wanted to be my same old self, still and again. As I write the book of my heart now, however, I find some truth to what they were saying. I am not entirely myself. It is indubitable that I have had a change of heart, and I confess that I want to remain faithful to that event, but it is not an event I ever expect to remember. Writing the book of my heart is such an act of fidelity, but it makes for a new me. By trying to remain faithful to a past, a change of heart, that is beyond my memory, I am giving birth to a new me, one that does not belong to the expectations of what I am because I can't remember it. A future opens in which I am not what I was and will not be what I am. That is also the logic of birth.

To replace my aortic valve, my heart was held motionless, inert in a state that endured long enough for the surgeon to transect the aorta, remove the failed valve, stitch in a new valve and segment of my aorta, and then close it all up. In fact, what I have come to see is that it wasn't mine that they operated on: *my* heart had to become *the* heart, detached from me and isolated. That's another thing that can be so disheartening about reading all this: not only that I learn how traumatic an experience it was but that *my* heart goes missing in it, precisely in order to save a future for me.

Everything I say in the course of writing about my heart, about me and mine, and what happened to it that afternoon is in fact something I learned about in the books and articles I read after the fact. I don't remember any of what I am saying they did to me. I don't find any of this in the great storehouse of memory that makes me who I am but in others' words. The book of *my* heart is blank on these matters while books of *the* heart are full of details and pictures. My memories of the heart I call mine come from elsewhere. They come from books I have been reading about the heart and heart surgery, and they come from others, those who wrote those books and also those friends and family who tell me the story of what happened as I woke from anesthesia. These books and those others might complete the story of my heart, but at the price of its being mine alone. It is, in fact, not uncommon for survivors of major surgeries to come to understand themselves in this way. Arthur Frank, a medical sociologist, tells of an author who was asked by a journal reviewer to revise his submission of an article that included reference to personal history. "In response, he subpoenaed and read his medical chart. He told me that he then understood for the first time, what had happened to him during his surgery and hospitalization."[10]

The fact that the effort to write the book of *my* heart has demanded that I turn to books about *the* heart and cardiac surgery means that what began as an effort of self-understanding, an attempt to tell my story as the story of my heart, has turned into a story told by others about the heart that is also mine. I can only write the book of my heart inauthentically, as it were, by reference to textbooks and expert journals where matters of the heart have become "objective," as they say, or an "academic" matter, susceptible to mechanical repetition, one like the other.

Telling my story has become less sincere, less heartfelt, then. I see that in the prose. It's dry, like the heart produced in the operating room, and distant, boring, even. There is for me some kind of comfort to be had telling the story of my heart this way. Telling it inauthentically buffers me from the pain of recalling it and from the worry of anticipating how it will end.

Its motions arrested, its self-directed beating stopped, so that it stands still for an extended period, the heart has been made available to surgical intervention and manipulation. The open heart can now be cut open.

At this point, different forms of open-heart surgery take different paths. A surgeon replacing an aortic valve will obviously make different cuts than will a surgeon grafting arteries that bypass blocked coronary arteries. Different replacement parts are called for as well, and different techniques for suturing them. In aortic valve replacement surgery, the surgeon transects the aorta just above the sinotubular ridge, the point where the aorta is rooted in the heart muscle itself, so as to expose the valve. Clamps and traction sutures are put in place to expose the surgical field, affording clear sight and easy access to the valve. A surgeon then uses scissors or knife and a vacuum sucker to cut out the damaged valve and clean up any debris. After the old valve has been removed, the replacement valve is put in its place. Dacron or nylon thread is sewn through the aortic annulus and attached to prefabricated loops in the sewing cuff at the base of the replacement valve. The threads are pulled tight, bringing the ring of the new valve to fit snugly, as seamlessly as possible in the annulus. Knots are tied, and excess thread is cut and removed. When the surgeon is sure that the replacement valve is seated securely, the aorta is reattached by sewing it back to its root in the heart itself.[11] It does not take long; most of the time in the operating room is concerned with stopping and starting the heart. The preliminaries to attaching the heart-lung machine can take several hours,

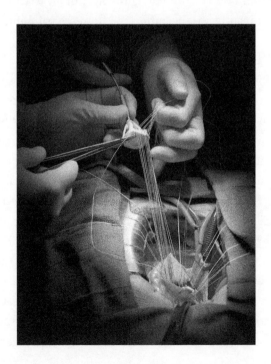

implanting the valve only about forty-five minutes from the time the aortic cross-clamp is applied.

All is well.

That, more or less, is the operation that gave me a future. I have tried to offer as straightforward and learned an account of the procedure as I can. Having such a heart is a bit discouraging to me who still wants to believe in the charming tale of a more precious heart harboring mysteries beyond what is seen "under direct vision" when discovered by the surgeon and his rib spreader.[12] It hurts to think about it happening to me. I can think about it, just that, as I have tried to do in the preceding pages, seeing it as the experts do, but knowing it that way from their perspective is different from thinking about it happening. Without its happening, just known, it is an abstraction, a heart without the fact of its existence being taken into consideration; that way, it can be thought about calmly, dispassionately, heartlessly even. But I can hardly read those pages about the heart without thinking about it happening and moreover happening to the heart I call mine, my existing, still existing, heart. How could I read otherwise than with my heart in it?

All is well.

*Really?*

# 2

## PRODUCING THE HEART

### A History of the Surgery That Gave Me a Future

Since our decision for aortic valve replacement surgery (AVR), I have discovered the obvious: there is a long history to which the procedure belongs. It gave me a future, one that would be greatly diminished had we not made the decision to commit to it. And it gave me a choice in which I was free to make a decision in a present that mattered, really mattered, because my decision would make a difference for a future that was open to me. That choice would not have been present had a tradition not made AVR available as a possibility. I knew nothing about the tradition when we committed to it, but without it, there would have been for me only the continuation of a past that soon would have had no future. Having chosen AVR, my future now includes its past, even though it precedes the beginning of my days. The history of AVR is therefore my history, too. It belongs to the book of my heart, in other words, the book I am writing. Any effort at self-understanding must include also an effort at understanding this history, appropriating it and owning up to it. I am its future.

Reading more about it, I have come to see that history as the disenchantment of the heart. It begins when the aura surrounding the heart decays, its sacred status profaned, as the heart that had been untouchable is touched by a few surgeons who are bold and dare to set their hands on it in efforts to repair it. What beat ceaselessly, without rest, and on its own is brought to a stand by techniques and devices that isolate and disembody it, rendering the heart open and available to experts, who knowing what to do with the newly produced object at their disposition, can do what they will with it to repair mine, in this sense like all the others. The condition for the possibility of my future is this demystification of the heart.

Popular accounts of the history of open-heart surgery often begin with either Dwight Harken on the battlefield of World War II; Ludwig Rehn at the hospital in Frankfurt, Germany, in 1896; or Daniel Hale Williams in Provident Hospital, Chicago, in 1893.

Williams, the first in the timeline of that list, was confronted with the victim of a stab wound in the upper chest, James Cornish. When weakness, fatigue, and low blood pressure indicated that Cornish's life was at risk, Williams opened Cornish's chest and discovered a wound in the sac surrounding the heart, the pericardium, which he stitched closed, "carefully timing the movement of his needle with the beating heart." Though first chronologically, this was technically speaking not open-heart surgery, since Williams did not lay bare the heart itself. It was nonetheless an important feat. It made him not the first to cut into the heart but the first to operate on one successfully.[1]

The first to actually penetrate the heart with his knife or needle, first, that is, in an effort to give a future, not take it away, is frequently said to be Ludwig Rehn. Jauhar takes this position in the popular *Heart: A History*, as do Larry Stephenson and Frank Baciewicz in the opening chapter of *Cardiac Surgery in the Adult*, a textbook used in medical schools.[2] James Forrester, the former chief of the Division of Cardiology at Cedars-Sinai Medical Center, also recognizes Rehn's significance, but he begins his highly praised book *The Heart Healers* with Harken in World War II for two reasons: first, Harken performed the procedure on 133 people, whereas Rehn, Forrester claims, did it just once; and second, Harken would record his achievements in the specialized journals read by experts who could build on his achievement. One is first, at least for Forrester, only when one's achievement allows it to be an actual beginning, and that means presenting it publicly in ways that let it be taken up by others and developed into a tradition. In only doing it once, Rehn did not begin anything. Williams, too, in not sharing his achievement with other experts by publishing his findings in the journals widely read by specialists, may have been original but did not begin anything— at least that is the reasoning that would make Harken first in the history of open-heart surgery.

Harken left his position in the Harvard Department of Surgery to serve the U.S. Army in London while Nazi bombs were ravaging the city. In June 1944, on what was also D-Day, Harken examined a dying soldier whose right ventricle, he discovered upon opening the chest cavity, had been pierced by a fragment of metal. To heal an otherwise healthy heart, Harken did what some say had not been done since Rehn just before the turn of the century: he put his hand on the still beating heart in order to preserve its life.[3] Forrester credits Harken with having thereby "dismantled the myth that the heart was untouchable."[4]

From there, Harken tied sutures in the heart in a circle around the bit of shrapnel lodged in it. This was made difficult by the incessant movement of the still beating heart, but Harken reasoned that "in the event of catastrophic bleeding, they could be pulled together, [becoming] an effective way of staunching the flow of blood."[5] He then made a small incision in the heart, and inserting a clamp to grab hold of the shrapnel, he pulled. The shrapnel popped out. As blood gushed from the now open wound in the heart itself, an assistant tightened the ring of sutures in an effort to staunch the flow of blood but to no avail. So Harken tried something new, as he writes: "I put my finger over the leak. The torrent slowed, stopped, and with my finger in situ, I took large needles swedged with silk and began passing them through the heart muscle wall, under my finger and out the other side."[6] From the time he cut into the heart until the time that incision was stitched closed, the entire procedure took only three minutes. Harken would go on to perform a similar procedure on the battlefield sixteen times, all of them successfully.

Those who attribute the beginning of cardiac surgery to Rehn in the hospital at Frankfurt, Germany, point to the case of Wilhelm Justus dying from a knife wound to the chest in 1896. Palpating Justus's chest, Rehn reasoned that the pericardial sac surrounding his heart was filled with blood oozing from a gash in the heart itself. Justus's heart struggled to beat against the pressure of the fluid-filled sac that now enclosed and pressed upon it. When he opened Justus's chest, Rehn saw his reasoning proved correct. Cutting the pericardium released the blood in it and revealed the heart itself with a tiny nick from which blood trickled. Rehn then did what Harken after him would also do: setting his hands on the heart, he stitched it with needle and thread. In Forrester's words, "He pressed his left index finger over the cut. The pressure of his finger staunched the bleeding. Justus's heartbeat continued steady but feeble. With his right hand, each time the heart filled Rehn placed a suture to close the wound. The bleeding stopped. . . . Rehn closed the chest."[7]

Rehn reports his operation in a lengthy article in the medical journal *Archiv für klinische Chirurgie*. A redacted and translated version appears in *Heart Surgery Classics*. It is the first recorded instance of cardiac surgery. Reading his report, I can feel the urgency of the moment in which he chose to do something for which tradition offered no guide, chose to act before all the information was in, to decide and be decided without the certainty of knowing it would work, because it had never been tried before. "Any surgeon can imagine the situation I was in," he writes. "Many facts could have been taken into consideration, but there was not enough time! . . . I was lucky to see the patient recover." The crisis thrust upon him called for a momentous decision made in a moment in which time was utterly lacking. Although there was nothing else to do, doing it felt illegitimate. Touching the heart, Rehn's act must have appeared to others and even felt to himself mad. Having tried all that was possible to a surgeon endowed with the best procedures offered by the institution of medicine, Rehn tried the impossible. The tension between the inner necessity to do the impossible deed of suturing a still beating heart and the public perception that such an action is rash, prohibited, mad, and doomed to fail is palpable to me in the apologetic, almost defensive nature of Rehn's report. "Because of continuous bleeding, I was forced to intervene in a case of a right ventricular stab wound. Trying the ultimate means to save the patient's life, I had to suture the heart. I had no choice. The decision was difficult, but otherwise, the patient would have exsanguinated."[8]

Regardless of the answer to the question as to who was the first to perform heart surgery, what appears clear to my inexpert yet very concerned reading is that the beginning of the tradition that transmitted AVR to me depended on a decay of the aura of sacrality surrounding the heart. That aura had led to a hands-off approach. The modern history of heart surgery would begin with the mad decision and profane act of violating the taboo against touching it. I can put my heart in the hands of surgeons today because over a century ago those madmen, those surgeons, profaned the aura that kept one at a respectful distance: they touched the heart.[9]

The taboo against touching the heart was common in the period contemporary with Rehn and Harken. This made it unique among other organs in the body in that by the end of the nineteenth century, "all [the other] major human organs, including the brain, had been operated on; the heart stood apart."[10] There were technical manuals and surgical textbooks in which procedures for operating on "the skeleton and its muscles, the mouth and jaw, the ear, the eye, the kidney, the reproductive organs, the urinary system, the intestines, and the rectum." But the heart "was still taboo." Its aura was spiritual or moral. The sixteenth-century surgeon Ambroise Paré, renowned as the greatest surgeon of the day, speaks authoritatively for many: "[the heart] is chief mansion of the Soul, the organ of the vitall faculty, the beginning of life, the fountain of vitall spirits."[11] One cannot cut into the house where the Soul dwells and expect the person to live.

But perhaps more important, the aura surrounding the heart was also practical in that nobody could produce desired effects when operating on it; it was therefore best left untouched. Its resistance to surgical manipulation was manifold: spurting blood obscured the surgeon's vision, rendering him unable to see it clearly and distinctly enough to operate effectively; shielded by the protective cover of the sternum, the heart was hidden and difficult to access; its incessant beat meant it was never at rest and therefore difficult to hold firmly enough for the desired operations on it. All this led to the professional taboo rumored to have been pronounced by the eminent surgeon, Theodor Billroth, whose authority among surgeons of the Victorian era was almost unquestioned. Hearing a suggestion that experimental operations on rabbits offered a technique that could be viable for stab wounds in human hearts, Billroth is said to have responded in 1883, "A surgeon who tries to suture a heart wound is sure to lose the esteem of his colleagues."[12] While debate is ongoing about the sense intended by Billroth, it seems likely he was advising his peers against undertaking a surgical adventure that was too difficult to hope for success. In effect, he was saying that, in 1883, touching the heart leads to professional death.

By the turn of the century, that taboo had been profaned. In 1907, Rudolf Haecker, a surgeon, wrote, "Since ancient times, the heart has been regarded as 'noli me tangere' [but now] the last organ of the human body has fallen to the hand of the surgeon. . . . In 1896, Rehn for the first time sutured a penetrating puncture wound of the right atrium in man. . . . The spell was broken. "[13] The ancient respect for the heart as a unique organ had fallen. Disrespecting the aura surrounding the heart and violating the taboo against touching it, the fathers of modern cardiac surgery treated it like every other organ of the human body. Indeed, they even treated it like organs of other bodies, for it was assumed to be like the heart of dogs and rabbits on which experiments had been performed in the laboratory: how else could these serve as models for its operation? "Rehn's and Williams's operations ushered in a new era," Jauhar writes, "in which the scalpel was applied to the most celebrated and elusive organ in the human body" (67). One could call that new era the era of the disenchanted heart. Freed of its spell, we handle it like any other organ or thing of the world, manipulate it as part of a project of repairing the body, remaking it as one whose defect I don't suffer, at least not insufferably.

When he profaned the heart by touching it, Daniel Hale Williams, in Jauhar's words, "did as much as any doctor in history to demystify the heart and advance the notion that it was a machine that could be repaired." The discovery that the heart could be repaired topples a famous pronouncement of Aristotle concluding "the heart alone of all viscera cannot withstand injury," a conclusion supported by Ambroise Paré, a renowned surgeon in Renaissance France, who declared that "if the heart be wounded, much blood gushes out, a trembling possesses all the members of the body . . . death is at the door."[14] It prevailed, too, at the turn of the twentieth century when Stephen Paget, a great authority among surgeons of the day, voiced it when he wrote in a widely used textbook, *The Surgery of the Chest* (1896), "Surgery of the heart has probably reached the limits set by nature to all surgery: no new method, no new discovery can overcome the natural difficulties that attend a wound of the heart."[15] The deeds of surgeons like Williams, Rehn, and Harken showed otherwise: the heart could survive its wounds. Rehn put it directly, "the feasibility of cardiac repair no longer remains in doubt."[16]

My AVR is premised on this, that the heart is reparable, constitutively reparable; heartbroken need not be the end of the story. The idea of living with something that is broken by fixing it challenges the aura of the original and the prestige of origins. Respect for that aura and awe at that prestige characterize religious man's attitude to the sacred according to the noted scholar of religion Mircea Eliade. The book of my heart does not belong to his tradition.

The immense respect of *Homo religiosus* for origins and the original state of things means he does not fix or repair them but longs for the original one, the thing as it was at the origin, in fact the origin of the cosmos, when all was whole, intact and, he believes, perfect. Commenting on what he calls the "archaic therapy" of *Homo religiosus*, Eliade writes, "What is involved is, in short, a return to the original time, the therapeutic purpose of which is to begin life once again, a symbolic rebirth. The conception underlying these curative rituals seems to be the following: life cannot be repaired, it can only be recreated through symbolic repetition of the cosmogony [the origin of the universe and all the things in it]." *Homo religiosus* is no repairman—and no cardiac surgeon. His world, a sacred cosmos, is not made of constitutively reparable things. Mine is. His world includes original things only, things that remain intact, whole and unscathed or else they are not real and do not belong to his world. Not so with mine: things in my world can break without being destroyed. Thankfully. For *Homo religiosus*, "sacred and indestructible" is a pleonasm, one frequently asserted. Rather than fix things, he abandons them when they break, seeking to return to the unbroken original in rituals that return to this sacred and indestructible time. Believing only in the irreparable, he believes broken things, too, irreparable in the opposite sense and therefore profane. He even encourages their destruction in rituals that "abolish profane past time" and "signify the end of the world," as is the case with the New Year's festivals Eliade delights in describing. The destruction they involve is in fact a ritual destruction of the broken, profane world and the broken things in it, so that *Homo religiosus* can return to the original time of original things, the sacred time where he has "vital forces *intact*," whole and unscathed. *Homo religiosus* would never accept a heart with sutures or seams, and a scar tells him only of the violation that profaned the once sacred integrity of the original now lost. There are no grades of sacrality: when the sacred breaks it is the profane; when it is profaned, it is not sacred.[17]

The fathers of the tradition of cardiac surgery disclosed an excluded middle, a place that I now live in and with: neither the intact, sacred heart nor the broken, profane heart, but the reparable heart. In the history they launched, a living heart need not be unscathed, a wounded heart still has a live future. But living with hearts defined by their reparability means that defective belongs to the possibility constitutive of what they are—and that they therefore need care, chronically and sometimes critically. This is not true of the sacred objects of *Homo religiosus*: their sacrality is either disproven or destroyed when they break. To some extent, then, he does not care for his sacred objects, for they are unbreakable and need no care. If the objects of his sacred world do break, he also does not take care of them, neither repairing them nor palliating them, but abandons them. I can't do that with my heart.

Having proven that they could touch what should not be touched and live, medical experts set out to apply their manipulations not just to critical emergencies but to the repair of chronic conditions of the heart. One of the first targets was congestive heart failure. This meant fixing structural flaws, most frequently holes in the septum or valve defects. The next wave of heroes in the tradition that is now mine would be found here.[18]

One, Charles Bailey, a contemporary of Harken, realized that the liberated act of touching it could be applied to the repair of a heart whose mitral valve was severely narrowed by scar tissue or other build-up, a condition known as *mitral valve stenosis*. The progressive blockage leads to congestive heart failure.[19] Clearing the obstruction could repair it. Bailey's procedure involved placing a circle of sutures in the outside wall of the left atrium, making a small incision in the center of the circle, just as Harken had done when removing shrapnel, and then, in an act I find incredible, inserting his index finger through the hole while tightening the circle of sutures around that finger to staunch the flow of blood. With the incision held fast this way and his finger inside the profaned heart, he would use that finger to, in Forrester's words, "blindly tear apart the scar tissue that held the leaflets of the valve together. Withdraw the finger while simultaneously tightening the sutures. Voilà, a cure of mitral stenosis."[20] A cure, indeed, but one that shows little respect for the aura or prestige of an intact heart.

Beginning in 1945 and running until 1948, Bailey's first four operations resulted in three deaths on the operating table and one the day following surgery. "A torrent, a gushing bright fury of blood" from incisions in the atrium, a "volley of arrhythmia" from ventricles quivering chaotically in response to his manipulations, and "torrents of blood flowing backward to the lungs" as the valve leaflets were not separated but shredded entirely by his blind fingers—this was "the carnage" he initially met. But after four deaths and the addition of "a small hook-shaped knife to the end of his finger" to facilitate clearing the valve, Bailey succeeded in June 1948 in repairing a stenotic mitral valve.[21] The patient, Constance Warner, lived thirty-eight more years, dying of respiratory complications following the contraction of herpes; her heart valve never failed again. Six days after Bailey's successful operation, Dwight Harken would perform a similar procedure on a twenty-seven-year-old man with mitral stenosis—successfully.

These profanations of the heart demonstrated that, as Bailey's obituary puts it, "the human heart could withstand manipulations which were previously considered impossible." It's not so fragile, so precious, or sacred that we need leave the heart unscathed. We need not be so deferential as to say "hands-off" in its presence. It can be cut up or torn apart—and with care, we can live on, live with a broken heart.

Merely touching the heart or even reaching inside it would not have been enough to help me. My valve was not stenotic but deformed and therefore leaky. Just cleaning it or loosening it up would not be sufficient to save me, it needed to be replaced. This was not possible when Harken and Bailey began their operations, for "the wall of the heart still presented a seemingly impenetrable anatomic barrier." To replace my aortic valve, the experts needed to "safely breach the anatomic barrier to the interior of the living human heart,"[22] cut into it, in other words, or at least transect the aorta so they could tear out the old valve and sew in a new one. I needed what the literature of the time refers to as "intracardiac surgery," otherwise known as open-heart surgery.

The next ingredient in the history that became the tradition of AVR therefore involved laying bare the heart and arresting its motions so that it stands still, open and inert. The heart brought to a stand this way before the eye and hand of the surgeon is an object that presents no barrier, no resistance, but is ready to be cut into.

Stopping the heart is not the hard part. Clamps or a tourniquet easily cut off blood flow to the heart and asphyxiate it, causing it like any muscle to contract more and more slowly, eventually not at all. The challenge is to stop the heart without that being the equivalent of death, how to produce, in short, a reversible cardiac arrest. This challenge was met by implementing a method and devising an apparatus that together produce *the* heart, an object open to open-heart surgery. The apparatus, better known as the heart-lung bypass machine, would set up the field of cardiac operations in ways that empower the surgeon to succeed.

Writing in 1954, John Gibbon, the doctor who many say "contributed more to the success of the development of the heart-lung machine than anyone else,"[23] described the dreamed-of apparatus this way: "The ultimate objective of my work in this field has been to be able to operate inside the heart under direct vision. An apparatus which embodies a mechanical lung, as well as pumps, enables you to shunt blood around both the heart and lungs, thus allowing operations to be performed under direct vision in a bloodless field within the opened heart." John Kirklin and colleagues, writing one year later about eight cases in which they used a mechanical bypass machine, also point to the important role that this apparatus plays in the methodic production of the object of open-heart surgery:

> The surgical treatment of certain intracardiac abnormalities in man demands accurate visualization of structures within the heart for a period sufficient to permit precise corrective measures. A method whereby this goal can be realized is the functional exclusion of the heart and lungs from the circulation of the patient by means of a mechanical pump-oxygenator system. . . . Use of this system established excellent conditions for precise, unhurried intracardiac surgery.[24]

The apparatus, the heart-lung machine, was the method to produce the object of intracardiac operations: namely, the heart seen clearly and distinctly "in a bloodless field" and holding still "for a period sufficient to permit precise corrective measures" desired by a surgeon. Time would stand still, a present held forever, or at least a very long while, for the surgeon who could operate on this object freely and "unhurried" by the nonpassing of any beat.

What Kirklin called the "functional exclusion of the heart and lungs from the circulation of the patient" rendered the heart distinct from other organs and isolated it from the whole of the organism, disembodying it, as it were. The need for isolating it is nowhere more evident than in the failures Bailey and Harken confronted when they tried to operate on valves of a heart still in motion and organically connected to the body as a whole. As

Forrester tells the story, it was a matter of losing control: they "punched a hole in the heart, believing they could control bleeding, desperately applied clamps to control it, lost control within seconds, then stood helpless in the face of exsanguination, facing a task as impossible as stemming the flow from a ruptured fire hydrant." A "torrent" or, in Forrester's words, "a river of blood" running out of their control obscured their vision and impeded their instruments, leaving the patient unavailable to their operations.[25] There is no controlling an embodied heart. The bypass machine, by diverting the river of blood around the heart and through a system of reservoirs, tubes, and pumps, effectively disembodies it. It produces a heart that barely bleeds, not exactly a heart of stone but a dry heart where the surgeon can see clearly and distinctly.

As Forrester observes, once the heartbeat can be stopped and circulation diverted so as to be maintained, "in principle, no form of heart disease was any longer beyond the surgeon's reach" (74). But while a still and empty heart is at the disposition of the surgeon, it poses challenges to other organs and tissues since they depend on the circulation of the river of blood. The biggest is posed to the brain. It can survive without oxygen delivered by blood for only about four minutes before suffering damage. This sets a narrow limit to the duration of the heart's availability. Most of the defects one hopes to remedy require the heart to be at the surgeon's disposition for a period longer than that. This is certainly true of an aortic valve replacement.

How then to extend the time during which the heart is present to the surgeon? The heart-lung machine answers that challenge, but it is not the only option that has been tried.

Charles Bailey used hypothermia—first in August 1952 when he attempted to repair an atrial septal defect, a perforation or hole in the tissue that separates the left and right atria of the heart. This disease was chosen because the repair is relatively easy: once the heart was exposed, emptied, and at rest, the procedure would involve nothing more than cutting it open and sewing the hole closed. But, though quick, it would take more than four minutes. Hypothermia extends that time. It reduces the body's metabolism and therefore lowers the brain's, and all organs', need for oxygen. Closely following research on dogs performed by Wilfred Bigelow, Bailey found in his own testing lab that a dog at 81° Fahrenheit could survive for twelve minutes without circulation to brain or heart.[26] In this way, the heart could be brought to a stand for a period that lasted long enough for quick surgeons to perform certain operations. Bailey proved it by repairing an atrial septal defect in a human heart in under six minutes. This first patient never returned to consciousness, but it was not because Bailey's heart repair failed. The patient died because air entering the circulatory system during surgery had blocked blood flow to the heart, bringing on ventricular fibrillation. Later that year, hypothermia would be used again in the repair of an atrial septal defect by Dr. John Lewis, who did succeed in bringing his patient back to the world.

To replace an aortic valve, however, the heart must hold still for more than twelve minutes. Where hypothermia falls short the machine succeeds. By extending the time during which the heart can be brought to a stand, it greatly enhances the surgeon's power to alter it. To do so, it relies on an external source of energy introduced into the no-longer-organic system of my now heartless body. That external source performs the function vacated when my heart is stopped. It can run, they assured me, forever, or at least as long as it remains plugged in.

But the stopped and empty heart also poses a problem for itself. Isolated and cut off from the circulation of blood, the disembodied heart is exposed to prolonged ischemia, an inadequate supply of blood and consequent oxygen deprivation, that puts it at risk of irreversible damage to the cells and tissue that compose it, known as myocardial infarction. D. G. Melrose and colleagues state the obvious in their paper "Elective Cardiac Arrest": "a most valuable contribution to this problem and indeed to the whole problem of intracardiac surgery would be made if the heart could be arrested and re-started at will, suffering no damage during periods of arrest and cessation of coronary blood flow."[27] The heart is at our disposition, they saw, not simply when we can elect to stop it but when we can do this so that we can also start it up again, "at will." "Elective cardiac arrest" is not killing it but imprisoning it, submitting its beat to our will, so that it can be given a future.

How then to protect the empty heart that rests in peace while the surgeon operates on it? Today this is accomplished largely by chemical means, most commonly periodic injections or infusions of blood-based cardioplegic solutions. Used in conjunction with hypothermic conditions, potassium-based cardioplegia lowers the heart's metabolic needs so that it consumes less oxygen and can therefore survive disembodied for a longer period without blood oxygenating it. These chemical means are the same ones used in execution by lethal injection. Cardiac arrest can also be induced through oxygen starvation by shutting off blood flow with a clamp, but that procedure is longer, slower, and riskier, a common danger being an air embolism that causes heart block or stroke when the heart is reembodied as the clamps are removed. Lethal injection provides better protection to myocardial tissue than death by hanging.

An early rival to the heart-lung machine was implemented by Walt Lillehei in 1954 when he pioneered a procedure known as "controlled cross-circulation." "Substituting the early mechanical oxygenators with human donors,"[28] Lillehei attached the circulatory system of a healthy "donor" to that of an ailing "receiver" by tubes installed in such a way as to bypass the heart of the recipient. This allowed the receiver to survive on blood oxygenated by the donor's lungs and pumped by means of the donor's heart with the assistance of a pump in the tubing mechanism. Controlled cross-circulation initially met with greater success than was being had by mechanical pumps and oxygenators, but shortly thereafter, Lillehei, too, had a run of failures, losing six patients in seven attempts over nine weeks. Added to that list was the case of a donor whose brain was so severely damaged by air bubbles in the tubing that she was left unable to care for herself. Lillehei, it was said by some, had a 200 percent victim rate. Serious ethical scruples were therefore raised against the use of cross-circulation.[29]

The modern heart-lung machine has proven, by contrast, both strong enough and ethically sound enough. It also has the advantage of being at the disposition of those who know how to use it. A machine, it can be turned on and off and adjusted at will by experts, empowering them to stop and restart the heart.

The first successful use of total cardiopulmonary bypass in an operation on a human heart was performed by Jack Gibbon in May 1953. Gibbon had been working on it since the 1930s, but on animals and unsuccessfully. His research and experiments demonstrated that life could be sustained on bypass, but he could bring only a small number back to embodied cardiorespiratory function and those only lived for only a few hours.[30] Gibbon's research was interrupted by World War II, but after the war he resumed his effort to engineer an effective cardiopulmonary device. The one he used successfully in 1953 was devised in collaboration with Thomas Watson, chairman of the board of IBM, who mobilized the company's engineers to the task.[31] After failing once, Gibbon performed the surgical repair of an atrial septal defect on an arrested heart that lasted twenty-six minutes.[32]

Stephen Paget's verdict of 1896 was overcome: "Surgery of the heart has probably reached the limits set by Nature to all surgery: no new method, and no new discovery can overcome the natural difficulties that attend a wound of the heart." That conclusion had been surpassed because we don't live naturally or just in Nature. We live in the world, and the world was now opened by the heart-lung machine. In this world, hearts have been brought to a stand well beyond "limits set by Nature." Having been born into the history of this world, I did not need to accept the gifts of nature as they had been given to me. What I am from birth, I don't have to be—that's the dream. . . . Or, is it this: because of what I am from birth, defective and constitutively reparable, I can't be as I am—that's the nightmare?

A reliable, effective heart-lung machine was an epoch-making technology in the history of the heart. It opened a new world with new practices, procedures, and ways to be. Albert Starr, founder of the Cardiac Surgery program at University of Oregon, goes so far as to distinguish historical periods of cardiac surgery in terms of it, "Pre-Bypass Procedures" and "Post-Bypass Procedures." These different procedures in turn call for novel devices. More specifically, Starr says, the bypass machine "introduced the surgeon to the problem of valvular heart disease, and by the end of the 1950's everyone was looking for artificial valves."[33]

A picture of mine follows. It's inside me as I write, but here it is before that, in the packaging that preserved it alongside all the other identical substitutes on the shelf where it stood on-call, at the ready, for the skilled and knowing hands of the surgeon who installed it. Installation does not sound complicated, once the heart has been brought to a stand and laid open, that is.[34] It's mostly a matter of stitching and tying good knots. The surgeon stitches sutures into the annulus at the root of my aorta and ties them through prefabricated loops on the valve, pulling tight to make a good seal but not too tight so as to tear the tissue of my aorta. A good seamstress could do it, they say.

The supplement, it seems, is not so dangerous anymore, and within a decade after the successful implementation of the heart-lung machine, artificial valves would be developed that would restore a heart's function to better than ever, make it young again. Strange categories I deal with now that my heart has been saved by its supplement. Am I older or younger? Closer to or farther from my birth, closer to or farther from death? Do I have a broken heart or one that is whole? Does the supplement to my heart confirm it is defective, and is the remaining defective now made possible by being in a state of repair? A thing repaired is broken, isn't it?

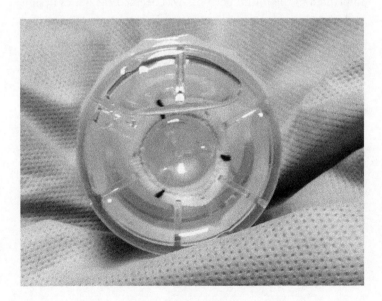

Several types of artificial valve have been developed. One of the first was by Charles Hufnagel in 1954. He placed a prosthetic valve in the descending aortic arch, not the intracardiac, natural position. This was not ideal as it made for ineffective management of regurgitation, but placing the valve in the natural position was not possible since he did not have cardiopulmonary bypass available to him.[35] Later, in 1960, seizing on the new world of possibilities opened by the bypass machine, Dwight Harken would place a prosthetic valve in the aortic position. Shortly after that, Albert Starr would implant a prosthetic valve in the mitral position. Though Harken did achieve long-term survival, his success rate was very low: four out of five patients died in the operating room or the immediate postoperative period. His failures had to do with valve design: the valve that had succeeded for Hufnagel six years earlier did not work for Harken owing to the hemodynamic demands of the aortic position and the pressures involved in flow. The valve used by Starr, though first implanted in the mitral position, was deemed the better design and fruitful for use in multiple positions.

That valve was developed by Starr himself in collaboration with Lowell Edwards, a hydraulics engineer who owned Edwards Laboratories in Portland, Oregon. The design problems they faced were twofold. First, could the artificial valve be attached with a seamless graft? A seamless graft would mean a perfectly secure fit, and perhaps just as important the absence of a wound where clotting of blood would risk the life of the graftee as her body tried to defend itself from what was in fact the life-giving artificial intruder. It was well known that embolisms were one of the leading causes of postoperative mortality. The second set of challenges pertained to the valve's longevity. Everybody knows that what has been repaired is reparable, which means forever susceptible to being in need of another repair. Could an artificial valve be built strong enough to withstand the forces that would buffet it over a lifetime of beating at somewhere around sixty beats per minute 24/7 until death do we part?

Starr and Edwards tried several designs modeled on a natural valve by implanting them in the hearts of dogs. These valves were failures. They then abandoned the effort to make a valve that copied the one nature gave and made a sort of ping-pong-ball-in-a-cage-like apparatus (akin to the metal basket that surrounds a champagne cork, only with a ping-pong ball inside it instead of a cork). These valves appeared to work, but it was difficult to tell how well as valve problems often become apparent only much later. Time will tell success in cases like this, and it is hard to measure a life still being lived. Several years after first implanting prosthetic valves, therefore, Starr and his group "began working at a frantic pace to analyze the results and develop changes in the valves. This resulted in many rapid modifications to the ball valve up until 1965–66." As is always the case in scientific communities dedicated to progress, researchers and engineers were trying to surpass results as soon as they were achieved. In this case, progress largely involved refining the design to favor longevity, ease of installation, and functionality. The ball was replaced with a disk then, in the late 1960's, with tilting disks and then with bileaflet valves, the first one designed by St. Jude Medical Co. and implanted in 1977.

Today the prosthetic aortic valve is a tricuspid version of the St. Jude bileaflet. It bears little resemblance to the ball-and-cage Starr first grafted into his patients. In fact, it is much closer to the one he first designed with Edwards, the one that failed, the one modeled on our native valve. Its leaflets were initially made only of synthetic materials, but beginning in the 1970s, valves made of cultivated animal tissue, porcine at first, then also bovine, were introduced. The benefit of tissue valves is lower risk of clot formation, while artificial leaflets are more durable. People who choose valves with artificial leaflets likely face a life on blood thinners, while those who choose tissue valves are likely to return for a new valve sooner. I chose the tissue valve and to watch vigilantly over expiration dates. My days are numbered.

Thus progressed a tradition of prosthetic valve surgery whose heir I have become. As Starr observed, "These valves . . . were an enormous success world-wide and engendered a tremendous amount of enthusiasm for valvular heart surgery. The reparative operations we had depended on before them were not reproducible and required a certain amount of artistry." But as it became a successful tradition, cardiac surgery became less of an art and more a matter of following proven procedures and deploying the right devices. At the beginnings of the tradition, it took a surgeon with gifted hands to do the work of manipulating a stenotic valve open with his finger, but the bypass machine and then artificial valve meant artistry yielded to technique, the singular to the reproducible. Of course, not everybody today can be a good surgeon, and there are some who have excellent hands, truly gifted.[36] I certainly wanted mine to be skilled and dexterous, good with his hands, but by the 1990s, Starr says, "Putting in a mechanical valve was just a matter of suturing it in. This was very reproducible, very subject to standardization, just the sort of thing that made surgeons comfortable."[37] Standardization, comfort, easily reproduced—the decay of the aura of the heart has progressed and now there are lots of surgeons who do lots of heart repairs, more or less the same all over the world. I enjoy the benefits of that progressive decay, that decay making progress.

# INTERLUDE

## ON THE SLAUGHTER IN THE OPERATING ROOM OF HISTORY

*January 2019.* When we decided for aortic valve replacement surgery, I inherited this history. I didn't know about it before that decision. I was just trying to save my life, and committing to AVR seemed the best way. Having decided for it, its history is now mine.

It includes a lot of carnage. Jauhar tells us that in the autumn of 1954, one season after the first successful open-heart surgeries using cross-circulation, "six out of seven cross-circulation cases ended in death. . . . [Walt Lillehei] performed forty-five operations with it, with twenty-eight long-term survivors, a mortality rate of 40 percent." The heart-lung machine fared little better: "From 1951 to 1953, eighteen patients were reported to have undergone open-heart surgery with heart-lung machine support. Seventeen died."[1] Before that, Charles Bailey, in 1948, had to watch four patients die before Constance Warner survived his finger reaching inside the atrium of her heart to scratch open her scarred mitral valve. This reckoning does not even mention the dogs, rabbits, monkeys, and other nonhuman animals that died, frequently painfully and often brutally, in sometimes savage experiments before human animals were brought to the operating table.

Carnage and death are attendant upon each of the moments of my history, then. History truly is a "slaughterbench," as the philosopher G. W. F. Hegel says.[2] And yet, it does seem that this slaughter belongs, as Hegel also says, to a progress, the progress that is modernity—in this case, the progress ending in aortic valve replacement surgery. After a steep learning curve at each of its epoch-making moments, the carnage shrank dramatically as the tradition developed. Five years after Starr began valve replacements, the operative mortality rate was under 10 percent. By 2015, the rate for all cardiac surgeons was close to 3 percent; in healthy patients, that number was even lower, less than 1 percent. Today, with standardized techniques and practiced procedures, a surgeon's operative mortality rate is less reflective of her skill and expertise than it is of her willingness to take on high-risk patients.[3] What is that if not progress?

I am not accustomed to admitting things like this. Having been formed in significant ways by the postmodern critique of the modernity in which history eventuated according to Hegel, I am prone to what Stephen Pinker calls "progressophobia." That is, I am accustomed to critical denunciation of modernity and to exposing flaws and unintended consequences in so-called progress. And yet, however much I find Pinker one-sided and single-minded, he is right that I, like the contemporary intellectuals he pillories, "prefer my surgery with anesthesia rather than without it," just as I prefer my heart with a prosthetic valve rather than without it. Here and now, I find myself unexpectedly calling "progress" what history made of this slaughter on the operating table.[4]

Many good people are unwilling sacrifices to this progress. History is heartless that way. Though each knew the risk they assumed when they submitted their beating heart, their trembling heart, their anxious heart doubtlessly trembling with fear of the unknown when they decided to be the surgeon's first operation—though each knew the risk, none wanted to die; each wanted to be the first to survive. As they were wheeled into the operating room, they may have found solace in the idea that were they to die, their death would contribute to the progress of history as the institution of medicine would learn from it, improve technique, and thereby make good of their bad end; but nobody wanted to redeem that ticket. The tradition that is mine is heartless when it lets us forget this.

Knowing the risk they ran and choosing to submit to the surgeon, these individuals cannot be called victims of injustice or bad intentions. I do not see oppressive and unjust forces operating on them. And yet there is evil in the progress to the good of AVR. The victims did not want to die. A friend pointed out to me that they were going to die anyway, of bad hearts that wouldn't have lasted much longer; there was no victim, then, she said, nor criminal, in what happened in the operating room. Yes, she was right, they were going to die soon. But they did not want to die today; I am almost sure they would have given anything to postpone it until tomorrow. Moreover, there was no reason it had to be the one who died who did die. It could have been another other or me. They were born too early. Arbitrary victims of birth, a congenital condition, or a disease acquired at random, sometimes children, not to mention the many, many innocent nonhuman animals, there was no reason they were elected to slaughter on the operating table of history, just ill-born and come too early. I, by contrast, am fortunate and well-off, having been born at the end of that history.

What I am calling the evil of their death belongs to history's heartless progress to a good, the formation of AVR. Evil? Yes, but progress, too. Progress? Yes, but with evil. Those evils become integral to what we call progress, and when so integrated, we don't call them "evil" but something else, a "sacrifice" maybe, in which the evil can be easily forgotten and heroism maybe even celebrated. In contributing to progress, the evils are said to be redeemed or justified by the good to whose production they now belong. They are no longer evils. Calling it a *sacrifice* instead, we elevate it to the noble status of having made something sacred (*sacrificium: sacer + facere*, to make sacred), a good, but I don't think anybody in this case wanted to be sacrificed. Let's keep in mind, then, that the evil became the good of a sacrifice from the perspective of the end, when we, its beneficiaries, know the result and tell a story in which the slaughter is part of a history that progresses toward a present good, such as AVR. They could not see that future or know the outcome as they were wheeled into the operating room. We, living in their future, are the ones who don't call their death an evil. Their death becomes a good only for me and those of us who, living after them, can tell it as part of a story. They themselves are not there to enjoy it when it becomes a good; the uses to which their deaths are put are made by survivors.

It is understandable that faced with the slaughter on the operating table of history, we would do our best to make some sense out of the carnage. All those books of the heart that I have been reading, Forrester's, Jauhar's, Morris's, and the rest, they can help answer the thoughtful person's question—What's the use? What good is it?—by showing the usefulness of the past in producing the present. They can help make some coherent sense of the madness by telling a story with beginning, middle, and end, a coherent narrative that assembles the pile of deaths into a story in which each moment is necessary as a step toward the next, redeeming it from the senseless contingency of time's barrage and the carnage attendant upon that barrage.

Have I, too, written a history that does this? Yes, I probably have, and in doing that, I probably have made my own case evidence for some sort of theodicy—my future justifying their death and providing some sense to it.

I do not want to have done that. I don't want the success I might enjoy let us forget the evil, the nonsensical deaths that we call instead sacrifices. All would be well if pain and loss were always and through and through sacrifice, but there is a dimension of it that is not—the death experienced by the others, those unique individuals who died their own death, an experience I cannot share. A secret, therefore, one each of them took to the grave. Only after the fact do they become sacrifices, maybe heroes, and as heroic sacrifices they are recollected for what they accomplished in dying (some small step toward AVR), but we remain oblivious to their suffering of death, a secret most personal and intimate. They take their secrets to the grave with the book of the heart they call mine, especially the secret of their death. I don't want the coherence of the story I told to let us forget these secrets we can never know, their death and all that was written on the book of their heart. I don't want to hide the uselessness and senselessness of their having suffered in secret their own death. I don't want to ask them to satisfy my need for a good story.

But I probably have. I probably have written a history in which the slaughter of the past becomes useful and appears necessary in progress toward the good of the present, my good. A more vigilant memory would remember the other death, the death of the other, unique and singular. Their dying their own death was not put to work for me but was suffered, purely suffered. Helpful to us, her death can be a sacrifice for our tradition, but it is useless in the life of that unique individual, a pure loss in the life that suffers it—uselessness itself perhaps. There is no compensation for her loss of all. A heart stopped, forever, a unique singular heart. It was not *the* heart that stopped there on the operating tables of Bailey, Harken, Lillehei, and the other founding fathers but a heart somebody called *mine*. The heart does not suffer death; *mine* does, and it can be hard to remember that I am not the only one who says that. A heart called mine, in fact many, stopped in order for us to know and produce *the* heart, object of a technique that would save many, many lives like the one I also call mine. Oblivious to the memory of those other hearts, lost in the slaughter, a heartless thinking of my history takes hold. Can I think otherwise? What would it mean to think about this history in a heartfelt way?

I confess to feeling a bit lucky. Lucky to be at the end of a history of aortic valve replacement surgery, for Hegel is right again, "history . . . is not the theater of happiness. Periods of happiness are blank pages in it." I am better off having had the good fortune to have come at the *end* of a history, the history of AVR, where happiness and satisfaction find a stage on which to appear.

In addition to lucky, I also feel something like guilt at my good luck: guilty in that I cannot repay those others for what I received from the heart they made available to me. The insurance company has repaid the doctors, nurses, and hospitals with money that has been agreed to be equal to what they gave (their time, expertise, equipment, space), but nothing sufficient, never enough, can be given to those who died for history to make progress ending in aortic valve replacement surgery: they died, lost everything, and I cannot give everything—or anything enough anymore to the dead. Sure, we make offerings to the dead, votives, flowers at the grave, and so on, but these gifts are never received and surely are not enough to compensate what they gave.

They gave up their entire life, the heart they called *mine*, and I received one. In return, I give . . . what? Flowers? A lit candle? Donations to the hospital or research center? Not equivalent. These words? I owe it to them to give something, and I am trying to now, but they don't receive equivalent compensation or even receive at all when I meet that obligation; they are dead. Giving them nothing, on the other hand, no words at all, would surely be worse; that would be a negligence that forgets their death, consigns it to oblivion.

Unable to give what I owe yet sensing that not to give at all is worse, what is left to do but give insufficiently, a giving felt therefore in guilt? A heartfelt memory of my history turns me toward the nonsensical evil of the loss of life, an evil from which I benefited. In telling this history of progress toward the happy days of AVR, I *should* feel a bit of sadness and some guilt if I have a heart. Contrary to a contemporary therapeutic mentality, a contemporary esteem of the easy conscience, guilt and sadness are not always feelings of which I should be cured but moods in which a heartfelt memory tells a story that remains mindful of the carnage and loss that is *not* transformed into the good of a sacrifice. It might sound cliché or like an excessive display meant to convince you of what I myself don't feel or believe, but it's true: when I am thoughtful and recollect the history of my AVR, when I have a heart, I do not grow reconciled to the slaughter but amazed at my undeserved luck and in my amazement feel sadness and guilt gnawing at me.

Sometime after I wrote these pages in January 2019, a friend recommended a slim book by Brian Doyle, *The Wet Engine: Exploring the Mad Wild Miracle of the Heart*. Reading it, I asked myself if there could be more than just guilt and sadness in the book of my heart.

Doyle was writing nine years after his son, Liam, was born with a heart having only three chambers, which is, in Doyle's words, "a problem, as you need four chambers for smooth conduct through this vale of fears and tears."[5] Liam had two open-heart surgeries before he was two years old and will need a transplant sometime in early adulthood when he outgrows the repairs, but he is, at the time Doyle writes, a normal nine-year old boy living a normal life. Not a day goes by, Doyle says, that he does not think of Liam "naked and torn open and heart-chilled and swimming somewhere between death and life; and . . . of the young grinning intense mysterious heart doctor who saved his life" (5). With these thoughts in mind, he writes a book like the one I am writing—one about the heart, how it functions, how it is repaired, how we came to know what we know about it, who was involved in that, and so on. His book is less technical than mine, more elegant and poetic, but like mine, his includes stories of the doctors and community of others who now make up his future. The tales he tells are more personal than the ones I do; they tell of doctors he met, one in particular, Dave McIrvin, whose story includes some pages on his mother, "Hope," and some in which we learn how much running matters to Dr. Dave.

Writing about his intentions in telling these stories, Doyle says,

> For years now I have wanted to try to write that most unwritable man down, to tell a handful of the thousands of stories that whirl around him like brilliant birds, to report a tiny percentage of the people he has saved and salved, and so thank him in some way I don't fully understand, and also thank the Music that made him and me and my son and all of us; and somehow it seems to me that the writing down of a handful of these stories will *matter* in the

world, be a sort of chant or connective tissue between writer and readers, all of us huddled singing under the falling bombs and stars; and more and more over the years I have become absorbed and amazed at the heart itself, the wet engine of us all. (5)

As a statement of purpose, this resonates with me. That it matters to those of us huddled together under the "falling bombs and stars" is something I want to believe about writing the stories I am telling, also that it can touch others and bind us together in a spirited song. More challenging to my sense of what I am doing with this book, however, is to see that Doyle conceives the stories he tells as an offering of thanks, a way to thank Dr. Dave, to thank the Music, and so on. He even goes so far as to call the book a "prayer of thanks" (6).

Doyle's book does anything but demystify the heart, disenchantment nowhere on his horizon. As he studies the heart over the years, reads the scientific books and the policy papers written by experts in public health, talks with the specialists surrounding his son—as he does all this, he only becomes more "absorbed and amazed at the wet engine of us all." His study induces a state of wonder in which, he says, "I sit my raggedy self down and write this lean book, as a sort of prayer of thanks that my son is alive and stubborn as a stone, that there are such complicated and graceful people as Doctor Dave, that there are such mysterious and holy things as hammering hearts, and that they power such mysterious and holy and wild things as us" (6). It would be nice to think of the book of my heart this way: a work of thanksgiving that issues from a state of wonder.

While I don't know if mine is that, *The Wet Engine* is. It concludes as such, with words that are common to a prayer of thanks, "Amen," several "amens" in fact: "so for this holy boy, and for great generous doctors like Dave, and all other miracles understandable and inexplicable, like wives and daughters and osprey and wine, I say amen and then amen and then again amen" (114). "Amen" gives thanks by affirming, saying yes, to gifts given: "so be it." Doyle makes saying it look easy here. How hard is it to seal with your "amen" and say thanks for obvious boons like "this holy boy," "generous doctors," wives, daughters, and wine, even osprey? Harder it is to conclude "amen" in a book of the heart that includes the heartbreak of having one. Doyle admits that such stories belong to his, what he calls "dark heart stories," alongside the "braveheart stories" he also tells. Friends die; people "take to bed with a gray heart," heartsick and never rise. A heart is broken so easily by so many things. He lists some: "a woman's second glance . . . the words I have something to tell you, a cat with a broken spine dragging itself into the forest to die, the brush of your mother's papery hand in the thicket of your hair" (85). A catalog of events that break the heart of anyone who has one is here included in Doyle's prayer of thanks. Even the boy he has come to call "holy" is in fact the broken boy who lives with an expiration date on his heart, anticipating a heart transplant to come. "Amen, so be it," Doyle says. How he can, where that comes from, I don't know.

As I read it, Doyle is inviting me to join him in this state of wonder from which a prayer of thanks issues, a state that religion often calls "contemplation." This invitation is made early on: "Let us contemplate, you and I, the bloody electric muscle. . . . Let us think carefully about the throb of its relentless tissue. Let us ponder it as the wet engine from which comes all the music we know. Let us contemplate the thousand ways it fails and the few ways it does not" (16). When we join him in contemplation, we are brought to see and stand before "the mysterious and holy thing" a heart is (6). The closer we get to it, the stranger, more mysterious, it seems, and the more we know about it, the more we are led to ask, "What is going on with it, I wonder?" As a contemplation, Doyle's book of the heart is not only an explanation, analysis, or assertion of information that tells us what the heart is and how we came to know all that about it; it does that to be sure: there is a lot of information about anatomy and physiology, how it forms in the womb, how much of the blood goes where, statistics relevant to its functioning differently in men and women. There are quite a few numbers. But through all that, *not* despite it or in addition to it, but through it, his book of the heart is, Doyle says, a way "to apprehend the miracle and study the mystery, and be agog and agape at what has been so wondrously wrought in the meat beneath the bone of your chest" (15). A contemplation, in other words, the book means to be an experience of this in wonder taking form in a prayer of thanks, "some strange act of celebration or prayer or testimony" (15).

I admire and respect that intention, but "prayer" is not a word I usually use to describe my doings or sayings. And yet, it might make sense, surprising sense, to think this way of the book I am writing. Am I offering "a prayer of thanks?" Is all this meant to be "in praise of the heart?"

I keep coming back to two things, though. First, my prayer of thanksgiving, my celebration of the heart, cannot escape the guilt and sadness that accompanies my opportunity to praise it. These feelings or moods are largely absent from Doyle's account. His thanksgiving is more joyfully innocent, I think, or perhaps innocently joyful. Some tell me that I should learn from him to keep in mind that it is a joy to give thanks, a joy then to write the book of my heart. They are right, but on that front, "my struggle" is evident. I do, however, speak of the history I am writing as a form of giving, words given to the dead others, words given to touch friends, students, family, children who are there with me, now, touching me. But I had not thought of it explicitly as a thanks-giving. Feelings of indebtedness and attendant guilt, of luck and contingency, set a different tone. And yet perhaps these do not contradict a thanksgiving, for what is giving thanks if not a recognition of having received a gift, something for which I am indebted even if the givers never intended me to be in their debt. The truth is, in this case, the dead didn't intend to give me or anybody else anything; they gave unwillingly in suffering and anonymously. Isn't there an element of luck or good fortune, and even guilt, then, in having the opportunity to give thanks? As for the feelings of guilt, no future will ever afford an opportunity to repay the debt of this past good luck, no matter how thankful I or Doyle is or how much giving he or I do. We both will remain forever guilty of not repaying what we were lucky to have received by accident from suffering givers. Feelings of luck and guilt therefore might not be so foreign to thanking. Perhaps the book of my heart *is* a prayer of thanks, even with its feelings of guilt and sadness? Maybe we shouldn't be so reluctant to take those feelings on, so eager for therapies that promise a happiness free of them?

The other thing I keep coming back to is this: Doyle's catalog does not include many reminders of those who were lost along the way, those who did not do anything except suffer death. Arthur Frank, a medical sociologist, says we should think beyond the heroes, that is to say, we should think about those who endured illness and maybe did not even succeed in surviving it. Or, if we want to keep the designation *hero*, we need to change the common sense of the word and say they are heroes but not by virtue of deeds or what they did.[6] Doyle does not go to the extreme of writing only about the heroic doctors. I am more guilty of that. His prayer of thanks has the virtue of being offered to ordinary doctors, men and women devoted to their jobs and the people in their care. But the gift to which he says amen is largely missing those who suffered in the history that gave his son a future.

There is a notable exception. A horse. A mare whose heart was cannulated as part of the Rev. Stephan Hales's early experiments (1714) into hemodynamics. When I read the words in Doyle's contemplation of that, I wept, big wet tears. I never found a passage like it in the accounts of the history of AVR. Neither Jauhar, nor Forrester, and certainly not the textbooks included something like this: ". . . ." I can't even copy it down.[7]

Thankful is indeed a better way to be. It's a joy to have the chance to give thanks, praise, and say "Amen." Maybe I shouldn't keep coming back to the dark spots. Thankfulness doesn't have to be just stupid ignorance. Doyle shows me that, too, but still, what of all the carnage?

It was, as I said, good luck that I came at the end of a history, and I am thankful for that. There was no reason aortic valve replacement surgery had to form, no necessity that it should have been the outcome of these events, and there was no original plan or initial design that was achieved by it. Rehn, Williams, and Harken were not thinking about AVR when they chanced, in a moment of madness, to put their fingers on a heart and thereby launch what would become, after the fact, the tradition that would give me a future. They were certainly not thinking about me, unknown heir to what they never knew they gave. Unplanned and unprovidential, not governed by a necessity, that history is nevertheless, by chance, a progress for me. A certain kind of piety might join with its opposite, a secular triumphalism, to tell me it was more than luck that AVR developed. They might say there is a necessity to these advances or a will active in them, that they belong to progress toward mastery of nature that is the definition and goal of the human spirit, for instance. Call it providence or call it reason, they say, you are wise to align yourself with its progress.

But I don't believe that. Did the story I tell here make it sound that way? When I am thoughtful about the history I have taken on and don't remain oblivious to the carnage, I see that I am lucky, just lucky, for it was contingency that made progress.

I am thankful, then, to have had the good luck to have come at the end of history. I did not have to be the first. In fact, what committing to the tradition does is make it such that nobody does it the first time anymore: my first time follows the model of those before; it repeats what has already been done, what is already known to work for others from whom I am no different, and so is much more likely to result in the desired outcome. Thanks to the tradition, we can minimize the carnage attendant upon beginnings—by not having to be always at the beginning. Whereas Starr performed valve replacement operations on only two patients in 1960, just fifty-five years later, by 2015, "we do about a hundred thousand heart valve surgeries in the United States, about a quarter of a million worldwide" each year. In 1954 Walt Lillehei was "the only person on the planet performing advanced open-heart surgery," but now the knowledge and skill has been passed on to apprentices, interns and residents all over the globe in institutions dedicated to forming skilled experts.[8] Research institutes, university hospitals, and professional journals provide important places where this tradition becomes actual and is actually transmitted.

Of course, for every surgeon there is a first time when she cuts an open heart and a first patient to receive her care. Each generation has to begin. Who really wants to be that first, especially that first patient? But if nobody does it a first time, no tradition would begin. And if everybody did it only the first time, the carnage would be unredeemed. The tradition depends on a first that it is designed to never have to suffer again. It takes a lot of failures, in this case a lot of permanently, nonelectively arrested hearts, before we come to the *first*.

But the truth is also that even if I was not the first, this was the first time for me. Even if the surgeon had done thousands, I had not done any. History is momentous that way even as it is predictable: from the surgeon's disengaged perspective looking at the global success, he knew it would work, but from my engaged and very concerned local perspective the future remained uncertain for me, and at bottom, I live life as me—which means, in this case, with all the anxiety of it being the first time. It wasn't just the heart on the table and in his hands; it was *also* my heart, a heart that wants to beat again.

I am, I said, lucky to have come at the *end* of a history. But what if I were to have come later? Would I be relieved of needing another valve replacement fifteen years from now? Or might my next replacement happen without cracking open my chest, without laying hands on my heart, without attaching the heart-lung machine—because it will be performed via a catheter, a technique called TAVR (transcatheter aortic valve replacement). The technique is being used as I write this in 2019. First done in 2002, it is included in the 2018 edition of a textbook for cardiac surgery specialists, where it is noted that TAVR is used for patients who are otherwise inoperable.[9] Even that restriction is lifting, however, as the procedure has met with more and more success, success that appears to be enduring success. TAVR means the end of open-heart surgery. There is still a supplement and an intervention, but life goes on while they work: they do not interrupt the incessant beating of the heart.

TAVR lets me anticipate a new epoch no longer using the epoch-making device that defined my era of history—namely, the heart-lung machine. This is a future age that might or might not be mine. When I reach the end of my heart's life, it is very likely I will not celebrate having been born at the end of a history but regret having been born too soon and dying early. What seems like the end will soon be surpassed, and something like what I said of others (had I been born like them, fifty years earlier, I would probably be dead) will be said of me. Children of the future will laugh that I ever even worried about an aortic valve replacement.

*Lexington, VA, January 8–February 14, Valentine's Day, 2019*

# 3

## CONCEIVING THE HEART

### A Pump at the Heart of Me

One of the marvels of the modern heart is that it can be stopped. The surgeons stopped mine, not to kill me but to intervene in ways that would give me more days and a better life. My heart no longer beat. Was I dead? Of course not. Mine is a secular age; even the theologians agree we inhabit secular times, the *saeculum*, in which nobody comes back from the dead, so if I am alive to write this now, I was not dead when they stopped my heart. Stopping it was not irreversible; secular death is. That's obvious, but the obvious should not always be passed over in silence.

An important operator of this marvel is the heart-lung machine. It is indeed epoch-making as Albert Starr said. Thanks to it, heart function can be maintained artificially. This means that in the epoch it holds open, my heart is not the seat of a unique, irreplaceable presence, the self or person; my heart can be replaced by a machine that does what it does while I continue to be. The heart can even be substituted with another without destroying the self as in the more and more frequently successful transplants. If machines like a pacemaker or artificial valve can keep the heart going and if heart function itself can be performed by a machine, then isn't the heart itself mechanical? Isn't it part of what the philosopher and early modern scientist René Descartes called "the earthen machine?"

The machine to which the heart is commonly likened is a pump. Sandeep Jauhar, a practicing cardiologist and bestselling author of medical histories, tells us that seeing the heart as a pump is in fact the foundation of training in cardiology and cardiac surgery. "From the beginning of my cardiac fellowship," he reports, "there was never really any doubt about how we were supposed to think about the heart. Despite its metaphors, the heart was best understood as a complicated pump."[1] However complicated, it operates in intelligible, predictable ways according to laws applicable to all bodily things and motions, including pumps, in this particular case. Faced with such an object, there are experts (doctors and surgeons) who can intervene (surgery), with technologically enhanced skill (the operating room and equipment it affords), collectively constructed knowledge acquired over time (medical school and research labs, libraries and teaching), and advanced devices (manufactured replacement parts). From the perspective of technical expertise, there is little mystery to the functioning of the heart. It's a pump and can be fixed like any other pump, until it can't.

The assumption on which my AVR rests, a heart is a kind of pump, has as its corollary the need relocate the self. If I was not given up for dead when my heart ceased to beat, this is because my living self or I is found elsewhere. Where? A neurosurgeon quoted in *Time* magazine (1966) tells me directly, as if I didn't already know: "The human spirit is the product of man's brain, not his heart."[2]

Reading, for understandable reasons, a novel titled *The Heart*, I found an inverse confirmation of this. The central character in the book, Simon Limbres, is declared dead in the first fifty pages

while his heart pumps on because it was attached to a mechanical ventilator quickly after he was pulled from a car crash. Reflecting on Simon's death, the author, Maylis de Kerangal, notes,
"the muscle continuing to pump is no longer enough to separate
the living from the dead. . . . The moment of death is no longer
considered as the moment the heart stops, but as the moment
when cerebral function ceases."[3] A machine, the heart can keep
pumping even when Simon is no longer—because he is found
in the brain, or in this case, is no longer there in the brain.
Now called "brain-dead," cases such as Simon's were once des-
ignated with the provocative phrase "living cadaver."[4] I was by
no means one, yet the concept that conditions my AVR (the
heart is a complicated pump) also gives rise to the living cadaver
as a meaningful possibility of being.

Such beings are useful medically for the practice of organ
transplants. A "cadaver" is suitable subject for donations as it has
no need for the organs that constitute its body, while the cadaver
must be "living" for the organs to be viable donations. Cardiopulmonary function, even assisted mechanically, assures the "living," while the "cadaver" is created by major injury to the brain.
That injury results from an accident, thereby relieving the need
for murder or factory farming of organ donors. Victims of car
crashes, like Simon, readily become "living cadavers" when
mechanical ventilators supplement organic function soon enough
after catastrophic damage has been done to the brain.

Along with the heart-lung machine, the law is an important
operator of the modern marvel of stopping my heart without my
being dead, as well as of this marvel's darker shadow, the living
cadaver. For it is in accordance with legal definitions that death
is declared even if that declaration is pronounced by medical
experts. In an epoch such as mine when the heart is a pump and
mechanical devices can maintain biological life by pumping in

its place, death is "determined by the condition of the brain alone." The "neurological definition of death" has replaced the more easily perceived and "commonsense notion of the end of life—a failure of the heart and lungs," confirmed ultimately by putrefaction, which anybody can detect without technological assistance.[5] Locating death in the brain and defining its moment as the cessation of cerebral activities, the neurological definition declares the legal and medical reality in which a heart does not provide evidence of life and death, conceiving it more like part of the "earthen machine" while locating the person in the brain where the moment of death can be seen.

The neurological definition of death was proposed in 1959, the year de Kerangal calls "the year death was redefined," by the French team Maurice Goulon and Pierre Mollaret. Speaking at the Twenty-Third International Conference on Neurology, they were the first to bring to public attention cases of *coma dépassé*, what we now call, in English, brain death. Mollaret had established one of the first modern intensive care units (ICUs) at the Hospital Claude Bernard in order to treat the large number of patients in need of respiratory assistance during a widespread outbreak of polio. Mollaret's plan included procuring as many mechanical ventilators as he could. The device proved revolutionary in that it enabled medical resuscitation of many failed respiratory systems, but it also produced many "living cadavers." Recognizing the challenge this machine posed to decisions in matters of life and death, Goulon and Mollaret proposed that such decisions be made on the basis of brain activity, not heart function.

Mechanical ventilators and heart lung machines had created beings such as living cadavers, but the need for a legal definition of death became urgent in the 1960s, when technological developments held open the possibility of using them as resources in the business of organ transplant practices. In a stunning book,

*Twice Dead: Organ Transplants and the Reinvention of Death*, Margaret Lock tells this story, noting two important moments in the coming to be of the neurological definition: namely, the formation of the Harvard Committee in 1968 and then, in 1981, of a special president's commission that called for a Uniform Determination of Death Act and proposed the neurological standard. Following the commission's proposal, the neurological definition was adopted by the American Medical Association, the American Bar Association and a majority of state legislatures. What Lock shows is that the neurological determination of death was the legal and medical response to the desires of medical practitioners, concerned populations, and moral philosophers, as well as businessmen, all of whom had an interest in legitimating and expanding the medical practice of transplant surgeries. Both the Harvard Committee and the President's Commission of 1981, Lock claims, shifted the criteria for their discussion about the location (brain or heart) and moment (cessation of electrical activity in the brain or stopping of heartbeat) of death away from "concerns about the *meaning* of death to defining it in instrumentally measurable terms."[6] Their aim clearly was to allow empowered agents to take action and intervene in the business of transplant practices, not to help us live and experience matters of life and death. Put bluntly, the practice of transplant surgeries required a legitimate business that could procure organs without the involved medical practitioners being guilty of murder: it needed a legally established category of "living cadavers."

What Lock implies but doesn't show directly is very evident to me: namely, that this is the age in which I have a pump at the heart of me.

The fact that a heart can continue to function even when, according to the neurological standard of death, I no longer am is the premise of heart transplant surgeries. In an important white paper published by the President's Council on Bioethics in 2008, the heart is described as an "autonomic system" that operates without reference to the central nervous system (CNS). The council goes on to write, "Even when there is no stimulus whatsoever from the CNS, the heart can continue to beat. This property of the heart, known as its 'inherent rhythmicity,' has been demonstrated dramatically by experiments in which an animal's heart is taken out of its body and stimulated to begin beating rhythmically again. It is also demonstrated by the heartbeat of an embryo, which begins before the CNS has developed." Margaret Lock reports that electrical activity in the heart can continue up to thirty minutes after death has been declared according to the neurological standard.[7] The fact that a heart beats autonomously without connection to the brain via the CNS means the one I call mine can also be yours. A heart is constitutively transferable, mine only by usufruct, as it were. Conceived as an "autonomic system," the heart takes up its dwelling place inside me contingently: it could just as well be in you. It lives on when it is given to another, and another lives when I give her my heart.

In matters of life and death, the brain speaks more distinctly than the heart to eyes opened in the age of mechanical ventilators and heart-lung machines. The President's Council makes this point when it says that the beat of a heart is one of the "automatic processes" that can be "continued by technological interventions." When hearts are thought of functionally, they are comparable to manufactured devices, like pumps. Being indistinct from a mechanical device makes the heart unsuitable to serve as the given for decisions about matters of life and death. As the President's Commission describes it, the ventilator "moves the lungs and facilitates the inflow and outflow of needed air . . . allowing the heart muscle to continue to function because its cells need oxygen to stay alive." This makes the heartbeat what the commission calls "a sign of life," but intelligent people are suspicious of signs, knowing that they don't speak their meaning directly and are likely to be confused with other meanings—in this case, a sign of mechanical functioning. That's why we turn to experts, the doctors and technicians who know how to read the signs—in Simon Limbres's case the doctor Pierre Révol, to whom death appears clearly and distinctly as he gazes intently at images of the brain seen on a screen: "yes, there it is, that's death," he says (27). Révol is not distracted by the beat of Simon's heart as he focuses his attention on the data shown on the screen and a picture takes form before him, an image of Simon's brain. "An abrupt vision, like a hard slap on the face, but Révol does not blink, concentrating on the body scan pictures and representations that appear on his computer screen," is how de Kerangal describes it. For an expert like Révol who can "read these images," the meaning is clear: "Simon Limbres's brain is dying."

Everyday opinion concurs with this relocation of our self from heart to brain. Most of us today suppose that the deepest mysteries of who we are will be uncovered by probing the brain, not the heart. Neuroscientists and cognitive scientists have more sway in public opinion over understanding ourselves than heart surgeons and cardiologists: the latter are plumbers and seamstresses; the former know what it takes for us to flourish. We fear that irreversible damage to our very self will be done by alterations in the function and processing of the brain, not the heart. Our fears are confirmed by cognitive impairments and diseases of the brain that alter our minds to the point where we no longer recognize ourselves nor others us. Alzheimer's and dementia sit only at the far end of a spectrum of negative confirmations of our sense that who we are resides somewhere in our head.

That popular opinion is voiced in scholarly books I was reading in the days, weeks, and months after surgery. Notably, Heather Webb, author of *The Medieval Heart*, says that we believe "single-mindedly in the exceptionality and superiority of the brain. . . . Once it was general knowledge that life ended when the heart stopped beating. Now we see hearts stop on television emergency drama rooms almost every night of the week. Usually, a doctor is able to jump start the unreliable thing. . . . Today, to establish end of life, doctors describe patients as brain-dead" (183–84). The heart having become just part of "the earthen machine," a pump at the heart of me, the brain becomes the place we look for evidence of our self, its life or its death.

The object of open-heart surgery, the pump Jauhar tells us he was trained to see, was not *produced* until sometime in the middle of the twentieth century by epoch making technologies like the heart-lung machine and legal, medical institutions like the neurological definition of death. But it was *conceived* well before that in experiments, interpretations, and debates between, among others, René Descartes (1596–1650) and William Harvey (1578–1657). They belong to the history we made mine when we decided for AVR as much as do the doctors and surgeons of the twentieth century. That is why I began to read and reread them.

Descartes is someone I had been reading professionally for many years, but Harvey was new to me. Based largely on experiments reported in his book *De Motu Cordis*, translated as *On the Motion of the Heart* (1628) (the full title is *Exercitatio Anatomica de Motu Cordis et Sanguinis in Animalibus*, that is, "an anatomical exercise on the motion of the heart and blood in living beings"), tradition has made him out to be the first conceive a modern heart. Two features are decisive in Harvey's conception. First, he sees the heart as part of a closed loop, a circulatory system confined within the body and in which blood alone circulates. Within this closed system, the motions of the heart can be reduced to those of a pump. That is the second claim. Both claims have become so common that few of us stop to think there was a time when somebody might have been surprised or skeptical upon hearing them, but that was so in Harvey's age.

Descartes, on the other hand, is not commonly known for things having to do with the heart, at least not in the circles I frequent. I knew him best for two assertions that many take to have inaugurated modern thought: the declaration *cogito ergo sum*, "I think, therefore I am," and the so-called Cartesian dualism, the strict separation of mind and body, thought and matter; taken together, these assertions are responsible, so the history of philosophy teaches, for identifying the self with thinking and thinking with self-possession. In my effort to own the history of the heart I now understand to be mine, I began to read a series of Descartes's letters and treatises I hadn't read before, or if I had, it was not with enough concern that they made an impression on me. In them, he sustains a polemic with Harvey on the matter of the heart. That polemic does not concern Harvey's enlightened efforts to explain the motions of the heart in mechanical terms but whether Harvey was thorough enough in that explanation. What Descartes objects to could be summed up in Harvey's invoking what he, Harvey, called "some inner animal [that uses the rest of the body] as dwelling place."[8] In having recourse to an alien presence or organic principle like a little animal, Harvey's account of the motions of the heart did not set the heart squarely within the "earthen machine" that was, Descartes said, the human body distinct from mind or thinking or self. To complete the demystification of the heart begun by Harvey, Descartes proposes a concept in which it is modeled on a bellows.

It is true, I know, that the model of the heart that dominates the science and medicine of open-heart surgery is the pump not the bellows. In that sense, Harvey is considered "right" and is more recognized within the tradition of heart repair than is Descartes. Yet it is also true that the modern heart is conceived more clearly in Cartesian terms, for the heart produced by the doctors and surgeons is not an animal inside us but a mechanical part of a mechanism.

Stopping my heart without declaring me dead is possible medically because of the heart-lung machine, legally because of the neurological definition of death, and conceptually because I am not found in my heart. This last point is Cartesian: I am found in thinking, he asserts. Today we are likely to say I am in my brain. Many of the authors I was reading identify this, too, as Cartesian, but that is a mistake: the Cartesian move is not to locate the thinking I am, the I that is thinking, in the brain. The neurological definition of death makes that move, but Descartes did not; he kept the two distinct. He is quite clear about this in a letter to Father Marin Mersenne, a Jesuit who was at the center of European intellectual life in the mid-seventeenth century: "One thing is certain: I know myself as a thought and I positively do not know myself as a brain."

That being said, the neurological definition of death does have a Cartesian condition: identifying the self with thinking and the heart with a machine. The next step was to locate thinking in the brain. De Kerangal alerted me to this. When commenting on the condition of Simon Limbres in *coma depassé*, she observes, "The moment of death is no longer considered as the moment the heart stops, but as the moment when cerebral function ceases. In other words: *I no longer think, therefore I no longer am.* The heart is dead, long live the brain" (31). There being no activity seen in the pictures of his brain, he must not be thinking, and (Descartes inverted) if he is not thinking, he is not; he is dead. This is also the logic that let the experts stop my heart without leaving me for dead. It rests on the assumption that we identify ourselves with our thought (Descartes), only then that our thought is located in our brain.

But it all supposes that we conceive the heart as a pump, and that goes back to William Harvey . . . and so do I, here and now.

Though tradition credits Harvey with having been the first to see the heart as a pump, this is not entirely accurate, for, as his English translator points out, Harvey "nowhere actually uses a word which may be literally rendered 'pump.'" That term comes from his, the translator's, effort "to present Harvey's thought in the current physiological manner."[9] Thomas Fuchs also points out in an impressive study that the only analogy in *De Motu Cordis* that is close to offering a mechanical model of cardiac motion appears just once and is more akin to interlocking gears activated by a trigger on a gun lock.[10] Fuchs reads *De Motu Cordis* in the context of the entirety of Harvey's work and is persuaded that even there Harvey explains the rhythm of the heart as a movement responding to the blood's natural movement to a center, the heart. For Harvey, Fuchs claims, blood possesses a natural tendency of its own, a "force" inherent to it, that activates the heart or triggers its beat. The heart moves mechanically, but these motions are not like a clock that runs by itself once wound; they are more like a rifle or other triggered mechanism needing to be activated again each time it moves or beats. "The triggering," Fuchs says, "cannot itself be interpreted in mechanical terms" (60).

Fuchs is persuasive in his account of Harvey's commitment to certain forms of vitalism—in fact, a reading of Harvey similar to Fuchs's prompts Descartes's own efforts to demystify Harvey's heart.[11]

These reservations noted, tradition and popular understanding are not wrong to trace the reduction of the heart to a pump back to Harvey, for Harvey will use "pump" in a few instances of self-interpretation (Fuchs admits this), and in *De Motu Cordis* itself, there is much in the language that invites seeing a pump in what he calls the heart. Perhaps the most renowned instance is this, translated as follows:

> Briefly let me now sum up and propose generally my idea of the circulation of the blood. // It has been shown by reason and experiment that blood by the beat of the ventricles [*pulsu ventriculorum*] flows through the lungs and heart and is pumped to the whole body. There it passes through pores in the flesh into the veins through which it returns from the periphery everywhere to the center. . . . It must therefore be concluded that the blood in the animal body moves around in a circle continuously, and that the action or function of the heart is to accomplish this by pumping [*actionem sive functionem cordis, quam pulsu peragit*]. This is the only reason for the motion and beat of the heart [*motus et pulsus cordis*]. (103)

What the modern heart does, the ventricles in particular, is push or propel blood, Harvey says. Its movements provide some sort of impulse or force. It pulses, like a pump.

It is not insignificant that what fascinates the observer of the modern heart is motion and forces, not eternal states. Setting out to explain the motions of blood in the body, in particular its observed circular movement, he looks to the heart, specifically its motions, and concludes that this motion (the heart pulsing) explains that motion (blood circulating). The modern heart is in motion, and its motion is a force that moves something else, forcedly, in a circle. There is no rest, short of stopping entirely. The world in which the modern heart is conceived is a restless one.

There is also a steady violence to the beat of this modern heart, a law-governed yet violent effect it has on its body's own blood. Fuchs puts it this way, "the circulation of the blood by no means appears in the *De Motu Cordis* as the quiet and 'natural' circular motion that, according to the ancient conception, belonged to the heavenly bodies. Instead, it has a violent character, which Harvey emphasized in contradistinction to the comfortable flow of humors in the old physiology" (47). The circles Harvey contemplates are not celestial, and the modern heart does not belong to a heavenly body. Blood, therefore, does not circulate calmly like the stars or other heavenly bodies of the ancient world but, in the modern world, belongs to an earthly body where even perfect, circular motions require effort and must be maintained by force, in this case the impulse provided by the heart and its constant motions.

Harvey vacillates, however. Exceptions to the forced motion of this earthly blood can be found elsewhere in his corpus, chiefly in later works where blood possesses something like an active principle or a purpose that energizes motions proper to it and works in conjunction with the actions of the heart to explain the interwoven motions of both. Fuchs also points to a few passages in *De Motu Cordis*. One appears toward the end of the book, in chapter 15. It arises in conjunction with Harvey's notion (dismissed today) that the force of the heart is "limited to the arterial side of circulation" (47). The heart not being strong enough to push blood all the way through the circuit but only up the arteries, how then does Harvey explain the venous return of blood to the heart? By suggesting, almost in passing, that blood moves *naturally* from the periphery or extremities to its resting place, the center, that is, the heart. Fuchs' point is well taken as a close reading of Harvey, but regardless of whether blood has no motion natural to it or, on the other hand, has a natural tendency to move to the center, in either case, it needs to be pushed or propelled out toward the extremities by a force: that is, it needs to be moved violently, even if regularly and predictably. That violence is provided by the pulsing beat of the modern heart, its pumping. "Blood requires force and impulse to be moved," Harvey says. "Only the heart can furnish this. . . . Force and effort, such as given by the heart, is needed to distribute and move the blood" (107). To see the heart doing the job of delivering the necessary violent blow that will push the blood on, one conceives it as a pump.

As I look at the modern heart conceived by Harvey, I see a worker, a hard worker, if not also a somewhat violent one, indeed one that exercises violence against its body's natural tendency to move toward a resting place. That is how it keeps me alive. A sort of law-governed violence conditions health, and if you don't have the heart for such violence, you will run down. All the movements of a healthy body are forced, and if you don't have the heart for such forced motions, you won't succeed in life.

The first study appearing in *De Motu Cordis* establishes this very point: the functioning heart works hard. It works actively by contracting, in systole, forcefully pumping blood out when it closes and grows small. Obvious to us today, it was not in Harvey's day. "The opposite of the commonly received opinion seems true," Harvey writes. "Instead of the heart opening its ventricles and filling with blood at the moment it strikes the chest, the contrary takes place so that the heart while contracting empties. . . . The heart does not act in diastole but in systole for only when it contracts is it active" (31). As Harvey notes, most of his contemporaries held that the heart works by opening, that it dilates to "work," when it swells and draws blood toward it. It is not entirely accurate to call this heart "active" when it "works": one could say instead it works when it relaxes. On this model, the motion of the heart belongs to a bodily system in which the parts are each regulated by "their respective *attractio*," the organs and tissues each possessing a "*facultas attrahens*" that determines the motion of the blood toward them (27). What to us, post-Harvey, looks like blood being propelled violently away from the heart looked to his predecessors to be blood moving toward what it is attracted to naturally, the tissues it wants to feed and nourish. This heart works attractively. Its attractiveness makes it swell. The picture is of a "relatively easy-going hemodynamics" (27), work that is not hard work but relaxed activity, where the motions of blood are like the ebb and flow of the sea, the stuff of meditative contemplation or poetic reverie.

Harvey's modern heart has little of the attractiveness that it possesses in these meditative and poetic models. It lacks, in Fuchs's words, "the *attractio* that had hitherto been a chief mover of physiological processes. Neither the arteries nor the heart move blood through suction, that is, active dilation, for expansion, Harvey says, occurs only passively and not autonomously" (46). For us, post-Harvey: an expanding, dilating heart is passive, not acting, and passivity is a failure. We need to act to perform successfully. The swelling heart that responds to attraction and attractiveness is a sign of weakness, reacting more than acting, lacking force. The modern heart is not like that: contracting to act, it propels the blood, actively forcing it to move. Like a pump, a hardworking pump. It's not very attractive, but it gets the job done.

Why does the modern heart move as it does? I have cited the answer Harvey gives. "It must therefore be concluded that the blood in the animal body moves around in a circle continuously, and that the action or function of the heart is to accomplish this by pumping. This is the only reason for the motion and beat of the heart." When the heart is a pump pumping on, "the only reason" that can be given for its motions is functional. Don't ask why a heart moves, ask about the function it fills, that's the reason. Or if you do ask why, answer the question in terms of its function. The motions of the heart are explained, or perhaps justified, by the function it fills, for its actions are equivalent to functions: "action that is [*sive*] function," he says.

Seen as such, Harvey's modern heart does not move because it feels something. A good student of mine, knowing I was writing the book of my heart but not knowing how deep I was in Harvey's work, recently pointed out to me that Thomas Aquinas also wrote a treatise titled *De Motu Cordis* and suggested that a good translation would be *On the Stirrings of the Heart*. He might be right, but in Harvey's case there is little question that it should *not* be rendered that way. The heart Harvey sees is a pump that is not stirred but effective in the performance of a function. Its motions are explained, or justified, or defined, by the part it plays, not by what stirs it. The "only reason" that can be given for the movement of the modern heart, Harvey says, is the function it fills within a corporate system—in this case, bodily circulation. That corporate system has need of a particular part to be played: it needs an engine to force blood otherwise at rest to move. Blood does not want or mean to make my tissues thrive nor does it know that it does that or was not doing that last August and September. Its motions are without regard for me and my wellbeing. Blood moves because it is forced on by the heart, and the heart pushes because . . . because it has a job to do in the closed corporate system that is the circulation inside my body.

The heart seen by Harvey has been reduced to its performance, action and function—more specifically, it has been reduced to action that is functional, and once it is reduced to functional action its performance can be assessed, quantitatively even, by measuring its effectiveness at this function. A dramatic decrease in the volume of blood ejected from the left ventricle, for instance, indicated that it was time to replace my aortic valve so that my heart could be restored to functioning as a heart should. The surgeon's operations did that. I am thankful for them. Making the heart function better, perform its role more effectively, the doctors see it as a pump with a function to perform, one they are confident they can repair when it breaks.

But I am having a hard time seeing it that way. Even though it no longer murmurs ominously and unhealthily like it did last August, my heart has not been entirely silenced. I still listen to mine, and that does not make me as secure as the surgeons and cardiologists appear to be about the object they know and produce. Most of the time when I think about my heart, it appears more like Harvey's "inner animal [that uses the rest of the body] as a dwelling place." There are times it roars so loudly it keeps me up at night, drumming an incessant, unrelenting and inescapable beat. I can feel it in my head on the pillow. There are other times when an unexpected swelling grows at the heart of me, and I have to sit up and catch the breath it threatens to steal away. My heart is not under my command even if I call it mine.

It doesn't listen to me so much as I it. My heart may as well be outside me, beating on without me within me. I admit to being horrified by Harvey's inner animal more than reassured by a pump.

As much as it is a struggle for me to adopt the doctors' gaze on a pump, it is also a struggle to look on with contemplative wonder. I would like to follow Brian Doyle and do so: "Let us contemplate, you and I, the bloody electric muscle," I remember he writes. "Let us ponder it as the wet engine from which comes all the music we know. . . . Let us contemplate. . . . Let us gawk. . . . be agog and agape at what has been so wondrously wrought." But what is so wonderful about having a heart, I ask myself when I listen to what comes from mine? I want to accept Doyle's invitation and join him in the wonder. Contemplative moments are glorious. I want to follow Doyle into his, gawk and dream with him and pass through the "amazing house, with its four rooms" then follow "the astounding journey your blood embarks upon as it enters the pumping station of your heart" (15–16). But I quickly come to what keeps me up at night, and I stop cold, frozen and stupefied in a now awful wonder. He lists it all: "Aneurysm, angina, arrythmia, blockages and obstructions, ischemias and infections, vascular and valvular failure, pericarditis and pressure problems, strokes and syndromes," ending with the horrifying "circus movement," what he calls "an electrical frenzy" (18), in which a disturbance of the electrical impulse that drives the pumping action goes awry, and the heart beats five hundred times a minute, putting it in an essentially continuous state of contraction. It can last up to ninety seconds before its continuous beat becomes beatlessness. No more rhythm. Dead. However wondrous I might come to see it to be, there is little joy in the thoughts that come from that wonder, and right now, truth be told, I am having a hard time even seeing it as wonderful.

That's what comes from listening to the heart I call mine. I am strung out, caught between the doctors and the poets.

Besides seeing the heart as a pump, Harvey's other contribution to the history that would eventuate in AVR is the discovery that blood circulates in a closed loop within the confines of an individual body. Observing that "in half an hour, the quantity of blood that moves through the heart is more than the quantity contained in the whole body," Harvey concludes that the only way such a volume could flow was if the same blood moved in a circle. Against those who accounted for the excessive volume by contending it was made by the body, in the liver from digested nutriment, Harvey countered that no human being consumed enough in so short a time to account for the enormous quantity of blood that his measurements calculated flow through a heart.

It seems to go without saying that the heart's "activity is limited to the interior of the body," but in Harvey's time this was a revolutionary claim. Its novelty can be felt in the introduction to *De Motu Cordis* where he spends what seems like needless effort to distinguish the circulatory system from the respiratory system. Numerous arguments are made, some rational deductions, many observations of anatomical functions—they feel excessive to my modern ears, but all are to the point of distinguishing the circulatory system. This distinction secured, nothing touches the heart.

Harvey's contemporaries saw something else. Relying largely on the authority of the Roman physician and philosopher, Galen, they saw a heart that was open, part of a system that breathed, one that took the outside in and put the inside out in the process of generating spirits necessary to animate our lives. In these systems, Harvey tells us, "The heart is commonly said to be the source and factory of vital spirits" (16). More than just functional action or active functioning, the medieval heart, a creative factory, created more than just motion: from this creative factory spring the spirits that animate the movements of life. The spirits generated in the heart were distributed through "arteries that contain and transmit them" to the organs and extremities of the body (10), thereby spreading the influence of the soul, *anima*, the life of the living, throughout the body. The soul animated the body, in other words, by being distributed in the spirits conveyed in and through blood, "ensouled life-stuff" Fuchs calls it (23), echoing the biblical use of the Hebrew word *nefesh*. To account for the difference between the voluntary and involuntary systems of living bodies, this model proposed that animating spirits were distributed through different channels of arterial transmission, one being controlled by the rational soul hence voluntary, the other by lower parts of the soul, hence not voluntary.

The heart-factory generates spirit in the way a volatile gas is released by burning a combustible. It requires heat, fuel, and air to produce the subtle spirits that animate life. The heat was provided by the heart itself. The fuel or combustible was the blood, which was made in the liver and conveyed to the heart by veins that carried it in that direction and in that direction only, no circuit or return trip since it was burned up in the factory of the heart or else exhausted in animating the body at the end of the tunnel. Finally, air was necessary for the combustion that volatized the blood and generated spirits like smoke or a gas. The air came from the outside, into the heart through a venous system open to the world in the skin and again leading only one direction, to the heart where it was burned up.

Crucial to this account is the conviction that there are what Heather Webb calls two "porosities" involved in the generation of spirit and spirited bodies. Regarding the first, Webb writes, "at the time Harvey was writing, most physicians were convinced that air entered the arteries through pores in the flesh and the skin,"[12] allowing for the in-spiration ingredient to spirit. A second set of pores, in the septum of the heart, allows the air in the arteries to pass from the right to the left ventricle where it mixes with blood and is warmed and volatized. At the end of this system of exchange, the used spirits, were exhaled, expired spirits, as it were, through the pores in the skin.

Porous, therefore, a body with a heart, was not in the world like water is in the jar or a chair in a room. At heart, you found yourself quite literally in the world, not just in your self or your body, and the world quite literally in you, not in-itself and over-against-you. This porosity was necessary to generating spirits and therefore to a person's resistance to the dispiriting tendence of the effort at living.

Both porosities vanish when Harvey demonstrates the circulation of blood in a closed loop. "Blood is to be found in arteries and blood alone," he declares, emphatically rejecting the heart's inspiration, as well as its expiration. Today we are more likely to conceive pores in the septum of the heart as a defect, atrial septal defect, we call it, and repair that heart with sutures that close them. That way, it functions better as a pump.

Turns out that the more porous your modern heart the lower the form of life you inhabit; the more open your modern heart, the less effectively it functions in the closed system. Harvey suggests this when in the concluding chapters of *De Motu Cordis* he uses the heart to sketch something like a hierarchy of animal life. Rank is determined by the degree to which the functioning pump establishes and respects the autonomy of the organism, secures its independence from the world.

Animals with low-level hearts (worms, for instance, or what we call cold-blooded animals), and, I would add, those with failed or failing hearts, are vulnerable to the world, porous, and less able to maintain themselves in a steady state—as when my weak heart fluttered and beat uncontrollably with excitement or worry in those days of August 2018. They find their heart changes with circumstances, its rate and pulse strength varying with the givens of the day: on cold days, the vital heat does not flow in them, their heart beats slowly; they lack vitality and make little effort at life, do next to nothing, and achieve even less. More developed hearts, ones that perform more effectively, according to Harvey's concept of the modern heart, are buffered from the mutability of the world. Fluctuations and changes in surrounding circumstances, the vagaries of the weather, for instance, or life's ups and downs, its twists and turns, do not stir such hearts— and if they do, the heart recovers on its own, easily reestablishes equilibrium, maintaining the motion of blood within the body so as to return the stability of its life. A steady reliable pump, keeping its own beat, is the ideal.

Along with this understanding of a heart's vulnerability or not, the sense of health, how we maintain it and recover has changed. A buffered self becomes the definition of health and health the definition of a buffered self. Belonging to an individual liberated from circulation with the world, Harvey's modern heart is not only index but also engine of this new-formed health. Just how it maintains health becomes clear toward the end of *De Motu Cordis* when Harvey conceives that engine in a sort of perpetual motion that lets it function as "place and source of life" (104). The opposite of life is death—which Harvey claims "is a dissolution resulting from lack of heat" (104). For a body to live, he says, heat must be spread throughout it. This vital and vitalizing heat is produced as an effect of the motion of the blood, for motion "always generates and produces heat, while in quietness it disappears" (104). Blood is put in motion, of course, by the motions of the modern heart. If these motions slow or grow quiet, blood stops warming the body. This is the case at the extremities, where, the force of the heart having diminished, blood's motion slows and "thickens from the cold and loses its spirit, as in death" (104–5). It is even more extreme in the cold when chilled hands, noses, and cheeks become "deathly blue" as the blood stagnates in them; limbs, too, become "sluggish and are moved with difficulty so that they seem almost deprived of life" (105). The lifeless limbs and extremities need to "recover heat" to recover vitality, Harvey says (105).

The modern heart is source of this recovery. Its pumping action restores health to life and limb by restoring motion to stagnating blood. "Thus the heart really is the center where this exhausted blood recovers life and heat," Harvey concludes. When the vitalizing flow runs down, the modern heart is strong enough to send blood back against the natural tendency to grow exhausted. Health rests on a sort of violence. The modern heart, a healthy one at least, never tires of this effort—until it stops. "As long as the heart is uninjured, life and health can be restored to the body" (105).

It seems right to me to say the heart is source of recovery. It takes heart for that. I am in the midst of learning so. Reading *De Motu Cordis*, then, I find what many take to be good news. At the heart of me, Harvey tells me is the source of my recovery. If I feel exhausted, the life force draining from me, good news: the perpetual motion of the modern heart, that busy pump at the heart of me, warms the blood that maintains health and vitality.

What might be better news is that recovery never need be an issue, since the perpetual motion of the modern heart means blood is perpetually warm. So long as the modern heart is in action, it never fails, blood moves, heat is distributed, and health maintained in a virtuous circle of motion producing heat-continuing motion. The modern heart becomes busy driver driving the internal motions that keep this individual moving in the perpetual motion of life, far from its collapse. Just keep moving.

Good news, then—and a prescription, too, a prescription I have always already filled. Keeping busy keeps you busy: that's the lesson of the modern heart, pumping away. Don't let its motions slow; they might not start again.

.

.

.

.

But hearts fail, they break. Mine did and will again. I am certain of that.

What, then?

# 4

# LISTEN TO YOUR HEART
## A Cure?

"Listen to your heart," they say, and it's good advice. I listen to mine a lot these days. It's harder than they make it out to be.

Most of my life, when I listened to it, I heard a murmur. That's what the doctors called it: a heart murmur; its beat was not clear and distinct. It would remind me of the uncomfortable certainty of an uncertain future, the promise of surgery one day contingent on the defector I carried within my chest. It was even more pronounced several months ago, before the operation. It was hard to think clearly through that noise. The thoughts that would emerge were hazy, blurred, mixed-up confused images of one thing tied to another and impacting all the rest, a cascade or avalanche of thoughts in which I would lose focus and get carried away in worry and torn apart in distraction.

These days, when I listen to my heart, though the symptomatic murmur is gone, its beat is a pounding I hear pulsing inside me. I hear it most undeniably at night. When I want to fall into sleep, it won't let me go. During the day we put our heart into all we do, and if it is a good one, we forget about it. Keeping busy and staying productive, engaged in the tasks of everyday life and all that is involved with them, I don't have to listen to my heart:

its beat slides into the background of the business of life, and I remain happily oblivious, obliviously happy, unmindful of its pulse. But at night, when I am in the dark, in bed, everything of the day fades away, all the familiar things and objects of my daily concern, all the usual tasks and projects to which I attend, all that I have put my heart into when rising to meet the demands of the day, it all slips away. When I hear nothing more of all this, then I hear it: my heart. My heart remains.

What will I do with it? Where can I put it? What will it take for it to go on? If I didn't listen to it, I would sleep and forget all about those questions, not give them another thought. But I can't. I can't not listen to it. *Can't not . . .* neither in the sense that I want to and have to listen, nor in the sense that I have to listen and therefore want to, but in the sense that it is not a possibility for me, not in my power to not listen. Undeniable. Irrevocable. Unrefusable . . . and at certain points, unbearable. In the dark, I can't not listen to it.

Some nights the pounding is so strong it hurts my eyes and I can't read. I turn off the light and try to sleep, but I cannot plug my ears to what shutting my eyes stops me from seeing: the heart beating inside me. Mine, it doesn't feel like it belongs to me. I don't feel it under my command even if I call it my own. It doesn't feel like something that listens to me but I to it. My heart may as well be outside me.

I can't be the only one to grow pale and horrified, stupefied and stammering, at the heart's incessant rumbling and alien beating without you within you, continuing without beginning or end that you know or will ever know. Another example comes from Paul Auster, the writer. Auster tells of a character named Blue who also finds himself delivered over to the undeniable beating of his heart. Blue has been assigned the mission of watching Black, who does nothing with his day, except read, write, and go for walks—more or less, the life of tending to my heart when recovering it these days. He takes it on devotedly. His days given over entirely to this nonproductive, inessential work that barely occupies him, Blue, like Black, finds

> this new idleness has left him at something of a loss . . . he finds that he has been thrown back on himself, with nothing to grab hold of, nothing to distinguish one moment from the next. . . . With the world removed from him, with nothing much to see but a vague shadow by the name of Black, he finds himself thinking about things that have never occurred to him before, and this, too, has begun to trouble him. . . . The beating of his heart, the sound of his breath, the blinking of his eyes—Blue is now aware of these tiny events, and try as he might to ignore them, they persist in his mind like a nonsensical phrase repeated over and over again.[1]

His world having become Black, Blue finds himself alone, with his heart, a shadow that does not disappear even in the dark. What thoughts come up then? What thoughts that never occur in the waking day of his active mind occur when he is left alone with his heart? Left at a loss in the darkened world and suspended business of life in it, what remains in his idleness is the beating of his heart. It makes no sense but beats on, a "nonsensical phrase."

When I listen to my heart these days with their nights, I can't ignore the "nonsensical phrase" Blue cannot put out of his mind, a beat within me that goes on without me. I often wonder, "When will it stop?" I don't want it to stop, but I wish it wouldn't go on. Life goes on without me within me. Difficult to listen to, this heart is hard to speak to. I hesitate even to speak *about* it, much less address it, monster that it is.

I am reminded again that William Harvey called it an "inner animal" that takes up residence in the individual.[2] Most days and nights, especially nights, when I listen to my heart, I think more of that than I do of a pump. It's not healthy-minded, but I can't help it. I am not always in command of my thoughts, especially not ones that come from the heart.

The "inner animal" bothered René Descartes, too—so much so that he would conceive its cure, a remedy at once inoculation and antidote for the heart whose beat carries me away when I listen to it. If I could think like he does, see the heart as he sees it, would I, too, be cured? Cured of my heart?

Descartes's remedy entailed demystifying the heart further than Harvey did when he conceived it as a pump, exorcising us of the little animal that shadowed Harvey's pump. Indeed, I am tempted these days to think of Descartes's entire philosophical career as reckoning with such a cure. He, too, sensed this. A couple years after the publication of the discourse that would make him famous as the founder of modern thought, the one asserting, "I think, therefore I am" (1637), and a couple years before the one in which he would follow up with the declaration "I am, I exist—that is certain . . . for as long as I am thinking" (1641), he admitted that settling the matter of the heart and its movements was indispensable to his thinking. He wrote to a friend and close confidant, Father Marin Mersenne, a Jesuit at the heart of intellectual life in the seventeenth century, "I am prepared to admit that if what I have written on this topic [the movement of the heart] . . . turns out to be false, then the rest of my philosophy is entirely worthless" (February 9, 1639).[3] What he wrote about the heart, I found upon reading more closely, was aimed entirely at its demystification, conceiving it ultimately as a bellows even more mechanical than Harvey's pump.

Though I had studied Descartes extensively in the past, I had never seen how important a concept of the heart was to his thinking. I knew him instead for having inaugurated modern philosophy with several famous doctrines: the equivalence of thought and being in the I; the strict opposition of mental and bodily realities; and the definition of truth as certainty. I knew him for promoting a form of thinking that was methodic, certain, and perhaps above all equivalent to myself, a way to self-possessed being or being self-possessed. Today we might call that form of thinking reasonable, good for problem solving. It's also not that far from popular ideals of a healthy mind.

What I find now, reading Descartes with my heart in mind, is that these claims serve and suppose a demystified heart. In the modernity inaugurated by Descartes, the thinking I am, the I that is thinking, is heartless, the heart thoughtless.

This discovery was disheartening to me. The surgery that gave me a future is premised on a heartless thinking? It supposes a heart that is thoughtless? Why would Descartes stake his entire philosophy on its heartlessness? Sure, it lets us be self-assertive and take charge of our hearts by repairing them or managing them so that they don't interfere with the workings of the everyday days of our lives. It might also let me sleep at night if I could get a grip on myself in thinking this way. But does thinking always have to be so heartless, our hearts always so thoughtless?

Descartes states explicitly the difficulty of Harvey's inner animal. "If we suppose that the heart moves in the way Harvey describes, we must imagine some faculty which causes this movement; yet the nature of this faculty is much harder to conceive of than whatever Harvey purports to explain by invoking it. What is more we shall also have to suppose that there are additional faculties which change the qualities of the blood when it is in the heart" (1:318). Descartes's worry is brought on by consideration of Harvey's faithfulness, or rather his perceived lack of faithfulness, to causes that explain. When the heart is conceived to move as Harvey describes it, Descartes objects, our thinking is led to refer to a cause that does not let us conceive "a full account of the bodily machine" (1:315), not all the causes of the motions of each of its parts are part of the machine that moves: the heart remains, a reality but one left out of the machine. Our thoughts thereby refer to a cause that does not explain yet still produces effects in the machine, mysterious effects of an occult cause.

When I read Descartes's accusation, I was taken aback. What could be more in keeping with a mechanical account of the body than treating the heart as a pump? Why would even Harvey's pump need to be demystified? Though surprising, what worries Descartes makes some sense. Ask yourself: What makes the heart beat when you think of it as a pump? Where is the cause of the heart's beat or the pump's pumping? What moves the inner animal to push on? Can you see distinctly, unconfusedly, the thing that would solve these problems? It sounds too willful, too spirited. Harvey has no intelligible answers to such questions, and without them, he cannot present a clear and distinct picture of an object, the heart. The heart, a lost cause at the heart of our picture of ourselves, makes for only a confused and hazy sketch of incomplete beings.

The answers I did find in Harvey's text only further Descartes's point. In a letter written in 1649 responding to Jean Riolan's belated disputation of his *De Motu Cordis*, Harvey speaks of a "pulsific faculty" that initiates the contraction of the right auricle. This phrase is used in explicit response to Descartes's proposal that the motions of the heart be explained by a cause external to them, with Harvey countering that they "come from

an internal principle." In *De Motu Cordis* itself, twenty years earlier, Harvey had already spoken of a "contractile element" that
is source of the active motion of the right auricle and of the
"pulsatile strength" that is "active" cause of the motion of the
blood.[4] All this, however, is precisely what Descartes means by
a faculty that is more difficult to conceive than the motion itself.
Harvey's account of causes does the opposite of solve problems:
it increases the mystery of the heart's pumping by referring to
active forces and faculties innate to the heart itself. Nothing is
cleared up by saying that the heart is the cause of its own motions.

From the perspective of a cure, it is also of little help. Harvey
leaves our lives dependent on a lost cause; we are at its mercy, at
the mercy of a little animal inside us—a fact that is never more
evident to me than at night when the one I call mine is beating
within me without me. A heart like that is not available to a medicine that wants to be effective in producing a cure that restores
healthy functioning.

A monstrous pump, then, this heart, mine, one that is so like
an animal. With "its special organs designed for movement," is
it alive or inert material? Soul or body? Does it act, or is it moved
to act? It is confusing, horrifying at times. A sort of monster
more than an animal, confounding as it does the living and the
mechanical. Thinking about such a heart makes for a mind that
is haunted, and the words I speak when speaking such thoughts
are vague and confused. No wonder Harvey, too, spoke in met-
aphorical language like "inner animal," and no wonder this "animal" should hold me in its spell. It's hard to get a grip on yourself or talk clearly when you are confused by a metaphor taken
to be real or by a reality made into a metaphor. Just listen to me
talk about it taking possession of me at night. When, in the dark,
I listen to that monstrous thing, I am often tempted to speak to
it in response, praying it, "Please don't stop!" or cheering it, "Get

up and go," or simply wondering, "What are you doing inside me? What, really, are you doing?"

The Cartesian remedy therefore advises me not to. Don't listen to that heart. Following that heart, you go out of your mind. It's a lost cause. Don't seek to find it. The healthy, modern heart, it promises, is much more manageable. If only I could keep my thoughts focused on it.

Like Descartes did. He even had a way to do so: what he called his "method." It is summarized in one of the books which has earned him recognition as the inaugural figure of modern philosophy, the aptly named *Discourse on the Method*. The book ends by deploying this method in an account of the heart's motions that unfolds in entirely comprehensible terms, making it, the heart, appear clearly as part of the "earthen machine" that is the human body distinct from the I that is thinking and the thinking I am. What interests me today is that the *Discourse* is the same book in which Descartes becomes the being of self-possessed thinking and asserts "I think, therefore I am." Sticking to his method, then, he could not only solve the problem of the heart's motions but actually be the being that was the solution to the problem that a heart appeared to be when thought about according to his method. Being cured, does that mean: "I think, therefore I am"? Is thinking this way Descartes's cure for the thought that can't not listen to the heart I call mine?

What does the heart look like when it is a problem you think about according to his method? Turns out it looks more like a bellows than a pump. Conceived by the Cartesian cure, the heart is a bellows whose motions are entirely unproblematic—a problem that is not problematic.

Here is how it moves. Blood enters the heart, drop by drop, from the vena cava. The heat of the heart, what Descartes calls a "fire without light," warms the drops of blood, like a furnace, rarifying them and causing them to expand as all liquids do when heat makes them approach closer to a gaseous state. The expansion of the blood causes the heart to swell, and as it swells, "the six little doors," the two valves opening onto the arteries, are stretched open, so that hot, rarified blood flows out of the heart to the rest of the body. As the heated blood exits it, the heart shrinks, then fills again drop by drop with newly entered blood that is still cold, waiting to be heated in the furnace of the heart, and the process of fermentation and overflow begins again.

It's that simple, that clear. No lost causes, no missing steps, nothing lacking from the explanation. "We do not have to suppose, in order to explain all this, any unknown or strange faculties" (1:318), Descartes says, no "inner animal" dwelling at the heart of me. Its motions reliable and predictable effects of causes, the problem is manageable for one who knows the laws that govern the operation of these causes.

Rendering the modern heart manageable and ultimately, some centuries later, reparable turns on Descartes explaining not so much how the heart moves as how it is moved, which means, for him, focusing on the problem of its swelling. It is significant that he puts his mind to the task of solving this specific problem, the heart's swelling, not its contracting. The swelling heart works in diastole, which is not so much an activity as a being acted on, stretched. This effect, he says, can be explained by causes.[5] It makes for a problem that is manageable as a predictable effect of other motions, such as blood filling it. It would be different if he focused on Harvey's contracting heart. Those motions look to him dangerously active; they are not effects but causes, and that poses questions that remain open to those who listen: Where does its beat come from? An explanation that refers to the thing being explained (pulsific faculties innate to the heart, for instance) does nothing to explain away the problem that thing is.

What attracts Harvey's thinking, Descartes says, is "the heart at the moment it acts," which is when he, Harvey, sees that it "becomes constricted." But for a thinking focused on problems of the motions of the earthen machine, this "acting" is nonsense, its beating a "nonsensical phrase." Where Harvey speaks of the "actions and functions of the heart," Descartes insists he has illegitimately added "act" to the list of what a heart does. Descartes speaks instead of "the causes of the motions of the heart," for caused motions are not actions but effects, predictable, law-governed effects, making for problems that can be solved.

The modern heart is conceived here, in Descartes's vision of Harvey's pump. It is the solution to a heart seen to be a problem. Even its swellings, especially its swellings, are a problem. But when our mind stays focused on the problem, a solution appears readily, a troubled thought is put to rest. Descartes can and does do all this. He constitutes the problem correctly, sticks to the problem methodically, and keeps his thoughts in order. Thinking like this, adhering to his method, he is the being who is the solution, not the problem, being cured of the troubled being I am at night when I listen my heart and what comes from it.

I sometimes wonder if Descartes listened to his heart. What did he hear of it? Did he not hear a stranger beating within him without him?

He must have heard it. The pages where he writes about the heart often reference it rising up to strike the wall of the chest where it makes its sound. He must have heard it, then, but it does not worry or distract him; he remains in command of his thoughts, and he orders them toward explaining the problem of the swelling heart. My thinking, following what comes from the heart beating within me without me, remains possessed by it, given over to what that heart gives me to think, especially at night. Heartfelt thinking maybe but not always healthy.

He must have heard it, for he took seriously the objection, raised by his friend the Dutch physician Vopiscus Fortunatus Plempius, that a heart continuing to beat after it has been removed from the individual in which it dwelled (vivisection) is evidence that it held some faculty of the soul. The observation was common, the interpretation subject of dispute. Eels, dogs, pigeons, rabbits, the hearts of all of them, had been observed beating on for some time after their shelter in the body had been exposed—that is to say, after the individual had been cut open and its heart removed. A gruesome gallery. Harvey talks about it; he even reports putting his finger on the heart of a vivisected pigeon, warming it gently until it beat again.

Yet even if he did hear it, Descartes is careful to demystify the phenomenon, offering Plempius not just one but five likely solutions, five explanations confirming the heart is body without soul or spirit. A first metaphysical argument relies on the believed indivisibility of the soul: how could that beat signal that the soul is housed in the heart if the individual has been divided and yet a soul is indivisible. The remaining four explanations all make for a heart seen clearly as part of the earthen machine. Demonstrating that it operates like a bellows shows, to put it simply, that the heart is thoughtless, has no intentions of its own, is not a little animal inside us, and is not endowed with a soul.

This is how you can a hear a heart and not worry or be distracted. Thoughtless and without intentions, it might beat nonsensically, its beat might be purposeless and unwilled, but the unintentional beating without him of the heart within gives Descartes no reason to fear, for he does not confuse the part of the earthen machine that the heart is with a living, thinking being and thereby make a monster of it—like I do. This is the second point for which Descartes is perhaps best known among the philosophers: the distinction between thinking and bodily realities, what has become known as Cartesian dualism. Again, in all the time I had been reading about it, I hadn't seen how it, too, is organized around the challenge of constituting correctly so as to cure the problem of the heart.

The advantages of keeping the heart clearly distinct from mind and will, I and thinking, are obvious. On one hand, I can think about it so as not to give it another thought. I remain free in the realm of Cartesian thinking. I can order my thoughts as I will. Someone in command of his thoughts, someone self-possessed who is equal to thinking the thoughts he has to think, is not rattled by what thinking has not put in those thoughts and is free, therefore, to think the next thought he wants to have, instead of what he might be led to think otherwise, by his heart, let's say, if he follows it. Descartes may very well have heard the "nonsensical phrase" that beats without reason, then, but the nonsense didn't disturb him. That's one thing you can do with a thoughtless heart. On the other hand, if I am concerned by what I hear, picturing it to myself as part of the "earthen machine" means I can assert myself over it, take steps to make it work the way I want it to. It might beat against me, but because it is conceived in thoughts that present it in a mechanical, not monstrous, order, it is all the more susceptible to a knowing will. That self-assertion is nowhere more evident to me than in cardiac repair.

Descartes may very well have heeded the advice "listen to your heart," then, but he listened to his heart so as to secure it and be secured against it, to guard it and be on guard against it. It's more like listening out for . . . the way we don't just look at something, contemplatively or appreciatively, but look out for it lest it happen to us. When I look out, things present themselves as a problem, which is not always a bad thing since problems have solutions—problems like those that were solved for me last autumn by the experts who *know* the heart's motions, and knowing that, *know how* to produce the effects we want to produce, and don't just know how but these days also *can* because they now control the tools, devices and chemicals that empower us to produce the heart we conceive. When you look out for the heart that has become part of the machine, you can manage quite well.

A lot of people think our heart is where we are truly ourselves. "Listen to your heart," they tell us. Doing so, we will know who we are, be constant and steady, authentic maybe. It, my heart, is who I truly am and so it will tell me what I really want. Listening to it, I remain faithful to myself and seek what makes me flourish because definitive of my true being. At least that's what I've heard.

But that's not what it feels like to me to have a heart. It sounds closer to what Descartes said was true of his mind, the thinking I am and the I that is thinking when cured of my heart. The heart I call mine, the one beating within me without me, still an inner animal, a spirited one at that—it gets in the way of that talk of self-possession, self-coincidence, and self-flourishing.

The one I call mine is more like the one I find in Augustine, the confessing Augustine that is. What are his confessions if not listening to his heart so that he can speak from it? And when he speaks from that place, he doesn't always seem to know what he is saying. He doesn't seem to comprehend what it is he hears when he listens to his heart: "I shall confess both what I know of myself and what I do not know," he says at one point in *Confessions* (10.5), and, more famously, "this then is my present state . . .

I have become a question to myself" (10.33). Listening to his heart, the confessing Augustine seems to be anything but cured.

Those who hold the popular conception that our heart is where we are truly ourselves also look to Augustine. They are not without reason, but the heart they see in him is different from the heart that draws me to him. The popular conception is voiced by Claude Romano: "Augustine calls 'heart' the place where the being of each man is disclosed to him in truth . . . the very place of my [selfhood]." Romano then cites a famous line from *Confessions*: "When others want to know what I am now in these days of my confessions, they have heard it directly from me or indirectly said of me but their ear is not at my heart, there where I am who I am" (10.3). My heart = where I am who I am; heart then as correspondence with my being, the place where I am equal to myself, fully me, that is, self-possessed; just what Descartes said happened in thinking. This is the foundation of the advice many offer when they tell us "listen to your heart": all will be well, they are saying, for, having found what's in your heart, the logic goes, you remain in possession of what can't be lost; true to your heart, you will remain steady and unshakeable for connected to the being you are, your self. You will flourish, realizing the truth of your being.

There is wisdom in such advice, but it does not come from the heart I listen to.

My heart may very well be disclosure of the truth of my being, but listening to this being most intimate to me means listening to a stranger. This is the case for Augustine, too, even after his conversion. Many readers would like to think that by this time he has taken the lessons of Christianity to heart, that he therefore has himself under control, that he has gotten a grip on himself. But, finding himself still in the world, finding he still has time, in other words, he continues on in confessing and tells of his present distractedness while praying a Psalm: it is a matter of the heart he has, still; he finds that he cannot take control of what he feels in his heart, for it runs off after the pretty sounds and sensuous melody that life has on offer and won't let him stay focused on more divine things, like the meanings of the words he knows he should attend to. "I find the singing itself more moving than the truth it conveys, I confess that this is a grievous sin. . . . This, then, is my present state. . . . I have become a question to myself" (10.33). His heart may very well disclose the truth of his being, who he really is, but that being is a question, hardly the solution to the problem that Descartes hoped he would be when thinking sticks to his method.

Along similar lines, Augustine imagines himself catching a glimpse of a curious sight, a dog chasing a rabbit in the wild, and worries he will be tempted to run after it in distracted curiosity. "Who can tell how many times each day our curiosity is tempted by the most trivial and insignificant matters? . . . If I should happen to see [this], the chase might easily hold my attention and distract me from whatever serious thoughts occupied my mind. It might not actually compel me to turn my horse from the path, but such would be the inclination of my heart; and unless you [God] made me realize my weakness . . . I should simply stop and gloat" (10.35). Again, it is a matter of his heart, where his weakness resides. Serious thinking does not follow distracted paths, but his heart might. He is not being forced to think along such lines, but his heart is easily led and likely to go down those paths; if he follows it, he will go astray. Perhaps worse, even if he sticks to the straight and narrow, he fears, his heart will not be in it; it will remain inclined another direction, tearing him apart even while going in the right direction.

Martin Luther, who launched the Protestant Reformation some eleven hundred or so years later, himself an Augustinian,

he too experienced having a heart to mean losing it, often moving in ways he knew it should not—as in the case of mourning
the death of his daughter Magdalena: "I and my wife should joyfully give thanks for such a felicitous departure and blessed end
by which Magdalena escaped the power of the flesh. Yet the
force of our natural love is so great that we are unable to do this
without crying and grieving in our hearts. . . . For the features, the
words and the movements of the living and dying daughter remain
deeply engraved in our hearts. Even the death of Christ . . . is
unable to take this all away as it should."⁶ He believes that Christ's
suffering for his sake has redeemed all loss, that his daughter has
gone on to a better place, that her departure is in truth a blessing
and he should not grieve, but he cannot take this lesson to heart.
He knows better, but his heart won't stop giving himself something else to think about. Heartfelt thinking, one whose thoughts
come from the heart he can't not listen to. Not even Christ can take
what I find in the book of my heart, Luther seems to say!

Possessed of a heart, the examples of Luther and Augustine
tell me, I am not possessed of myself. "My heart" is too much
for my self. That is not the heart Descartes conceived. Instead,
"My heart is where I am *whosoever* it is that I am."

The formulation comes from Augustine (*Confessions* 10.3). The
place where I find myself, in truth, my heart, Augustine says, is
"where I am whosoever I am [*cor meum, ubi ego sum quicumque
sum*]." It is as if I am most myself there where I don't know myself
or how it will turn out, who I will be and what will become of
me. I have already cited this line, in a more common English
rendering, "my heart is where I am what I am," but "Where I am
*whosoever I am*" is closer to Augustine's Latin words and experience. It states the strangeness introduced by having a heart—
strange both in that my own heart is unfamiliar to me and also
in that it will vary, given over to the twists and turns of a life lived

in mutability, making me whoever it is I will be each time. Augustine does not say "*sum qui sum*." He does not say his heart is where I am what or who I am. That is the divine way to be. It is how the divine identifies itself to Moses when Moses asks its name at the burning bush in the biblical book of Exodus (3:14). A being who speaks from the heart does not speak that way; having found his strange heart, he finds, "I am whosoever I am." A heart is not a "what," and having one, I too am never what I am, self-possessed or equal to my own being. That would be to be God, who does say, "I am who I am [*sum qui sum*]." I, however, will be, so long as there is world and time and I have a heart in it, forever estranged from the divine life. Strange being that I am with a heart.

Descartes did not want to listen to a heart like that one. He saw the one I and you call mine as a problem, and seeing it as a problem, he was able to solve it. It's not that different from how Brian Doyle imagines the renowned surgeon Francis Fontan saw the hearts of his patients when he operated. "Surgeons tend to think of their patients as problems to be solved," he says after meeting Dr. Fontan.[7]

This is an important ingredient to the cure for the heart: see it as a problem. Descartes had a way to see it as such: "the method." Sticking to the method, he could be delivered from the problem it led him to see: that monstrous little animal becomes the object we know so well, the heart. Perhaps a heart becomes a problem, then, when thinking becomes self-possessed and aims to cure what is not. Putting it that way, I sound like I am getting the sequence backward, putting self-assertion before problems arise, but there is truth to that backwardness: self-assertive thinking sees problems everywhere, everything as a problem, challenges for which it is the solution.

This is clear to me when I look at the development of Descartes's philosophical thought. Beginning in a work titled *Rules for the Direction of the Mind*, it culminates in the *Discourse on the Method* and *Meditations*. When he eventually becomes the being who says, "I think, therefore I am" (*Discourse*) or declares "I am, I exist—that is certain. . . . for as long as I am thinking" (*Meditations*), he realizes, actually realizes, comes to be, the form of thinking outlined in the *Rules*. Those rules, it turns out, were instituted as a way to constitute a world of problems, so that he could have ideas of their solutions, eventually be the being of that solution, which he finally realized when he asserted "I think, therefore I am."

The fact that self-possessed thinking is tied to a world of problems whose solution it is must be understood within the framework of what I consider the third distinctive characteristic of Descartes's heartless thinking: the desire for certainty. From the outset of his philosophical biography, Descartes wants more than to know truths; he wants to be certain that the truths he knows are true. Being-certain, that was his ambition, one that would last a lifetime: he wanted to be the being that was certain of the truths he held; they would be permanent that way. Wanting to be certain, Descartes takes everything to be a problem—everything, even the truth. I admire the existential concern, being-certain transcends a mere speculative interest in truths he knows, but my experience has been, especially of late, that such existential concern will not be accomplished in certainty of the kind he seeks.

The truth of things appearing problematic, the solution Descartes finds is to adhere strictly to rules that govern the operation of his thinking. In particular, he assumes, you can be sure that what appears truly to be the case is certainly the case if the idea of it was produced by following specific rules. Those rules are formulated in his "method." It is elaborated over the course of the *Regulae*, then repeated some ten years later in condensed form in the *Discourse on the Method*. The being who thinks according to his method (according to the *Rules*) is the one who says *Je pense donc je suis* (the *Discourse on the Method*). What is hard for me to forget now is that this is also the being cured of a heart you call mine.

It is not insignificant that the method Descartes discovers is a method for *thinking*, rules for managing thoughts in an orderly way, where "orderly" means according to the order of thought. It seems obvious, but it could be otherwise. It could be that thinking responds to an order outside it, arranging matters under consideration according to the dignity or value of the being concerned; theology might do it this way. It could also be that thinking is ordered by what is appealing, calls to it, luring it on or attracting it as in desire; an aesthetics of beauty, not one of critical judgments, might do it this way. In such cases, matters would appear in truth when thinking is sensitive to orders received, when our thoughts follow these orders—as if I were listening to my heart and the thoughts that come from it. Descartes's methodic thinking refuses to follow orders of anything other than itself. Following the method, it listens only to itself.

The title of the work in which the method was first set forth, *Rules for the Direction of the Mind*, suggests it is a guidebook of sorts or a user's manual for thought to think certainties. It turns out that there are eighteen rules to which his thinking adheres to form certainties. The later *Discourse on the Method* condenses these, bringing them down to four. They are recognizable as rules for problem-solving. Those rules, Descartes says, are these: (1) Form judgments based solely on what is "present in the mind so clearly and distinctly that there is no occasion to doubt it"; (2) "Divide each of the difficulties I examine into as many parts as possible"; (3) "Direct thoughts in an orderly manner, by beginning with the simplest and most easily known objects in order to ascend little by little, step by step, to knowledge of the more complex"; (4) Make complete and comprehensive enumerations or chains of knowledge that "keep to the order required for deducing one thing from another" (1:120). So widely accepted today has the idea of thinking as problem solving become that these rules appear commonsensical. It's difficult for us to imagine how else one might put thought into practice. Anything else would not be thinking, but what . . .? Daydreaming? Delusional? Possession by spirits or demons? Listening to your heart?

What interests me now is not so much the specifics of the rules but the fact that Descartes had a method that let him see problems, everywhere and only . . . so that he could inhabit a world of problems solved. When he adhered to the method, he would be the being who is the solution to the problem, the self-possessed being, a being-certain—also and therefore the being cured of a heart.

Here then is the Cartesian remedy for my sleepless nights: If I follow his method and approach the heart as a problem, my thinking will be self-possessed, and I will be cured of a heart I can't not listen to; or else, starting the other way, if my thinking remains self-possessed, I will think methodically, and I am exorcised of the monstrous heart. Either way, I am cured of the heart that worries me . . .

. . . but neither way is something I am up to these days. Mine is a telling failure, one that tells me that it takes an operative will to stick to the rules of thinking and be the being that is the cure for my heart from my heart. This is a will I still do not always have the heart for. Try a little harder, one might say, a lot harder if you need to, put more effort into it, but that again calls for the heart I don't have. My will, rooted in the heart, is not equivalent to my command, not always summoned so readily, not always prompt and eager in its effort, and my thinking therefore less self-possessed, less certain and more hesitant, vacillating.

Descartes's method is a supplement to efforts rooted in the heart. Like all supplements, it strengthens, in this case strengthens the heart of a willing thought and thinking will, but also like all supplements, it lets the heart be replaced. Follow the method, not your heart. A lot of people have mastered this. I meet students, for instance, who have become very good at following the rules that produce the application that gets them into the best college, then makes for an "A" paper at that college, then produces the résumé that will get them the perfect job after college. They can also be very good at following the rules that produce the composed and collected, or else enthusiastic and committed, self-presentation that will win any and all of the above success. But their heart is not in it, and you can tell—it does not come from the heart. They are often left succeeding in a life that their heart is not in.

When that happens, when thinking does not come from the heart but from the method, the heart becomes a problem. . . . and problems have solutions, final solutions that eliminate the problem: in this case a thoughtless heart, ultimately, I fear, a disheartened one. I exaggerate, of course, but maybe less than we'd like to admit.

# CURED OF THE CURE:
# SPEAK TO YOUR HEART

*March 2019.*

*Much of my reading and writing of late has been an effort to own up to the heart that belongs to the history that gives me a future. In the Cartesian explanation of the heart Harvey saw, the modern heart was conceived. This is the heart that by the end of the twentieth century could be produced: doctors and surgeons did so in the operating room where they gave me one. It is the heart I have to live with, repairing it, for the rest of my days, and having to live those days, it is the heart I have to have. Accepting it is the only way for me to have more days up ahead. The cardiac surgeon Albert Starr once wrote to that effect: "one of the important elements in this history [of the modern heart] is the total acceptance by the patient of a life-sustaining artificial device. . . . Artificial valves were the first lifesaving implantable devices; their long-term fate was completely unknown and yet patients accepted them gratefully. . . . Life was sweet, even though it was dependent on an artificial device."[1] Maybe. I can accept the pump they see at the heart of me, but perhaps more is required to say "life is sweet" than just accepting the modern heart and its history? It takes heart, another heart besides a disheartened one, to face the days that remain.*

Having accepted the heart conceived by Harvey and Descartes, then produced by the doctors and surgeons, I am nevertheless having a hard time getting back into the days of my life. Where do I look for the heart to recover those days?

The Cartesian remedy is impracticable, especially at night when my lost heart can't stick to the method, and it's not even desirable: I don't want a cure of the heart that leaves me heartless.

Harvey's pump pumping on also seems of little use.

He tells me that the heart is where the exhausted look to recover and regain vitality, that the modern heart is strong enough to put the exhausted life force back into motion. He spreads the good news of the modern heart, a prescription for health: its perpetual motion keeps us moving through the days; so long as it moves, it keeps moving and keeps me moving.

But I wonder from I where I sit these days, and I sit a lot these days living on with my failure of a heart—I wonder how spirited this modern health is. After all, its health and vitality depend on motion, forced motion moreover, not on generating spirits by being part of a creative process. It is not concerned about spirit or spirits, high or low, inspiration or expiration. It's true that buffered from that, it never has to think about giving up the ghost, for definitively dispirited, all that motion doesn't seem to have one. And it's also true that buffered from that, it is less dependent on others, who might be withholding, or on things out there in the world, which might be broken.

The modern heart may very well be "place and source of life," as Harvey calls it, but what kind of life is it? The life of what kind of being? One whose hearty action has been reduced to function, one whose performance is measured by quantitative assessment regimes, one whose successful performance comes at the price of creating nothing? I wonder if all this perpetual motion belongs to what will soon be, if it isn't already, a heartless being. It takes a certain kind of thinking, heartless thinking, to get on with all that. Was that what Descartes realized, to be that kind of being? I don't know if I have the heart for it. I don't know that I want to have the heart for it. A cure for the heart that cures me of the heart?

The recovery that many of my post-Harvey contemporaries promote might not be one at all. It certainly does not speak to where I am. A healthy modern heart is never lost or at a loss. What sense is there to the recovery of something that is not and never is lost? A modern heart looks to me less like source of recovery and more like what lets us avoid having to confront the question of recovery. It belongs to somebody who always already has the heart for it and so doesn't need it.

It is as if we with our modern hearts, being self-possessed, think about *having* the heart to face our days without ever thinking about *finding* the heart for facing our days. We think about *taking heart* without asking after what might *give the heart* we take. We think about the heart as something we *possess* without experiencing the *need* for that possession or the *neediness* that is possessed by one.

But one loses heart. I did. I do. And hearts also break. Mine did. Mine does. They get tired and need to stop and need to get going again before they stop finally.

When lost or brokenhearted, the very idea of having the heart for life becomes difficult and enigmatic. Much of the talk about recovering my days sounds to me like it is talking about it to the healthy, a case of supposing I possess the heart I am being told how to find. The virtuous circle of circulation's perpetual motion then sounds like a vicious one. Those who find themselves outside it are a bit skeptical of the circle's good news. Not that it is wrong or false, it's good advice to remain active and stay productive, but we are unsure how the good that it is certainly known to be can also be a good in the case that is mine.

Not taking the Cartesian cure and holding Harvey's heart to be of no avail, I will have to listen to my heart, for it's not going away and I don't want it to, and I will have to speak to it, since it's not going away and I don't want it to. I don't experience it as a problem that can be solved so much as a question that has to be addressed. I can't solve it, but I can't ignore it. I have to speak to it. Speaking to the monster I listen to is the only way to inhabit that strung out state of being in the incurable position of having a heart I call mine.

We listen to others. We speak to others. Sometimes we say we know them, but we don't: that's why we speak and why we listen. We do not have a clear and distinct idea of what is before us, so we listen to what comes from the distance and speak to it, or we speak to the distance and listen to what comes, or does not come, back from it. We don't have to speak or listen when we already know. Approaching the world by speaking to it is the way to enter that unknown land—very different from approaching the world through an idea you have and have formed correctly in which you already know something in advance of hearing it call to you. It's easier to be certain that way: you never come across strangers.

When I listen to my heart, then, I admit it as an other at the heart of who I am, whoever I am. And if I speak to it in response, urging it to press on, asking it who it is, I enter into that strangeness, a strangeness at the heart of whosoever I am. Self-possessed beings do not speak to themselves; it's madness. Or perhaps put better, self-possessed beings speak to their selves but not to their heart. Listening and speaking to my heart, then, not myself, I am in conversation with a stranger, an other that poses questions. A self, by contrast, listens and agrees with me. The correspondence I exchange with myself is perfect.

Owing to this perfect self-correspondence that is the disheartened self, we never need address our self, never call on it or to it. It's not that we don't speak to ourselves—the phrase "I said to myself" is common enough, but it usually means I am saying something I know and comprehend, not posing questions or responding to a stranger. Who ever says "O' my self" when they aim to take on the truth of their being disclosed to them in an honest confession? Nobody. That is because we, myself and I, correspond perfectly. Being disheartened, or else oblivious to the heart, might be the price we pay, or the condition for, this perfect correspondence.

If we don't hear "O' my self" open any speaking to myself, we might hear somebody say "O' my heart," a bit like "O' my soul," but anyone who says that sounds archaic or old-fashioned, unfashionable or untimely, for nobody talks to their modern heart: why would you, it's a pump or bellows, steady and reliable, manageable; when it breaks, it does not need to be addressed with words of encouragement or cheer, it needs a good technician with the right tools and chemicals to treat it, an expert surgeon or someone who can write a prescription, or for those who prefer DIY, a technical manual and a user's guide available at the local bookstore or checkout line of the supermarket. Saying "O' my heart," you would sound like the Psalmist of the Bible: who spoke to his soul this way, "Why are you cast down, O my soul" (Ps. 42:11, 43:5, etc.); and like Augustine in whose confessions such an address, O' my heart, is implied throughout but is also explicit as when he loses heart for pressing on in the difficult work of meditating on the intersection of time and eternity, death and life, and, beginning to lose it, exclaims, "*Insiste anime mea.* Press on, be resolute, o' my soul" (11.27).

You would also sound like Zarathustra, "Zarathustra, the godless" (283), the protagonist of Friedrich Nietzsche's infamous book *Thus Spoke Zarathustra*, his "gospel for all and none," who spoke to his heart, crying out, "Up with you now, come on, my old heart!," similar to the Psalmist and Augustine in this regard. A strange, motley genealogy . . . of which I find myself part. It's an unlikely community and an odd parentage for anyone to confess, as if the marriage of Augustine and Nietzsche could issue anything.

# 5

## "UP WITH YOU NOW, COME ON, MY OLD HEART"

I often hear the lost heart that needs to be found in the phi-losopher who many say stood closest to the edge of the abyss of modern life, Friedrich Nietzsche. Nietzsche struggles to find the heart it takes for a spirited life in this world and some-times can barely manage it. Heartfelt, his writing is, I find, heartening. Many students disagree. Most find him dishearten-ing, to say the least, and are more likely to think of him as cold and cruel than heartfelt.

Diagnostician of nihilism, its history as well as its present and future forms, Nietzsche saw purpose, unity, and truth withdrawn from the universe, he saw that "the aim is lacking, why finds no answer." In such a cosmos, the "only reason" a heart beats, to put it as William Harvey, conceiver of the modern heart, did, is to produce the effect of motion, to keep us busy in what Nietzsche thought of as "the blindly raging industriousness" of modern life.[1] The good people around him, Nietzsche saw, they with their modern hearts, never seem to tire of being productive, never seem to admit exhaustion or look up from their toil in longing for anything other than success in the business of life become a business to manage. For such a life, the heart is a pump, a hard-working reliable, steady pump. It is a heart that can be had without any questions being asked, and it doesn't even know that about itself. It took Nietzsche to tell it so: "you don't have any idea why you are doing this" or, in his words, "Why? finds no answer."

Nietzsche did not give modern hearts any answers, however. He simply called it to a reckoning with its truth and asked it to find what it would take for it to go on. Students don't always see this about Nietzsche: he did not make the modern heart that way, he told it its truth. What they also don't see readily is that he cared for it, tried to take care of the modern heart, help it find, and take, heart for inhabiting the days that remain. Like the minister students might meet in their religions.

When I read Nietzsche, I cannot escape the impression that he finds his heart failing him, he loses heart, has to find it, has to recover it so as to recover ("convalesce" is a word he uses frequently), and finding it loses it again as if the heart he found was precisely a lost heart. I try to convince students that this makes a difference. The example I point out comes toward the end of the work Nietzsche always identified as closest to him, *Thus Spoke Zarathustra*,[2] when the protagonist, "Zarathustra, the godless" (283), "Zarathustra, the advocate of suffering, the advocate of life" (328), says to his heart, "Up with you now, come on, my old heart!" (389).

Students don't get it. He's godless, they say, and that makes him unlikely to have beliefs or values that will motivate or guide his actions. The rallying cry will never succeed. It doesn't sound very heartening to them. He is the advocate of suffering, they say, and he believes that makes him also the advocate of life. They can't imagine anything more disheartening than to hold suffering and life to be bound together, to believe life something to suffer, suffering essential to life. Why would I find that heartening, and why especially be reading him now when I look to take heart?

These students have not shaken the common view of Nietzsche as one of the loudest voices of modern nihilism. Nihilists, they are convinced, do not address matters of the heart. Most of the students take Nietzsche to be heartless and cruel, the best illustration of this being for them his unrelenting and vociferous, frequently mocking, critique of the value of pity. It is not pity speaking when he offers his heart the encouragement he does: "Up with you now, come on, my old heart." The students are right about that. The ethic he teaches is one they take to be cold and hardhearted, as when he champions the virtues of the beast and the warrior over and against those of the common and the slave. Proclaiming himself teacher of the Overman, his mission in life, they say, is unfeeling, insensitive and must come from a heart of stone. Why would I ever consider looking to such a hardhearted man, heartless even, when tending to matters of the heart? What could he teach me about living with a heart? Good questions.

I am drawn to Zarathustra's cry, I tell them, as an exclamation that comes out of the situation to which it speaks. "Up with you now, come on, my old heart!" An effort to find heart if ever there was one and so an effort that implies a lost heart. And yet, this seeking to find the lost heart is spoken to the heart that is his own, the one he calls *mine*, "my old heart." It is, in other words, an effort spoken from the heart he has lost to the lost heart he has. This is recovery speaking, one I can understand, a circle that turns in ways that make sense to me. It speaks to the heart *out of* the experience of having lost heart, and so *back into* the experience of having the heart to lose—having a lost heart.

"Up with you now, come on, my old heart!" It sounds like a command, which it is, but it could also be a prayer, for prayers are like commands but ones spoken by those lacking power to bring it about. Born from the loss of the things it addresses, what are the words "Up with you now, come on, my old heart" if not a heartfelt command made from need and neediness—a heartfelt prayer, in short, to a heart that cannot be commanded to do what it is not given to do, the heart he calls *mine*. No guarantees but he gives it a try. He prays it to get moving.

I read much of Nietzsche's writing as a prayer like this. Essays, in both senses of the word: short writings from life, and also tries or attempts, at taking heart. Writing, he listened to his lost heart, spoke to it and, out of this experience, spoke from it—or wrote from it, composing what often sounds to me like the book of his heart.

*The Gay Science* includes one of my favorite examples. Nietzsche opens the fourth part with a declaration of intent that belongs to what resembles some kind of recovery program: "I want to learn more and more to see as beautiful what is necessary in things. *Amor fati:* let that be my love henceforth! I do not want to wage war against what is ugly. I do not want to accuse. . . . Someday I wish to be only a Yes-sayer" (§276). Nice sentiments. They are well-known lines in Nietzsche scholarship. Students spend hours debating their meaning and writing papers about their truth, their validity, or their significance in the context of Nietzsche's work, but what interests me now is their genre: they are resolutions, a resolve to some kind of health (to be "a yes-sayer," "*amor fati*," to see things as beautiful, to overcome the feelings of hate inside me, and so on). Nietzsche, in fact, presents them explicitly as New Year's resolutions. Here are the first lines of the paragraph: "*For the new year.*—I still live, I still think: I still have to live, for I still have to think. . . ." It's a new year, he finds himself still alive—and one has to hear not just a little astonishment in him as he says that, an astonishment to which I can relate. Finding himself still alive, as I do myself, he needs to recover the days of the year to come. Finding himself still alive, he needs to begin the days again, a new year. In that neediness, he looks to his heart: "I shall say what it is that I wish from myself today, and what was the first thought to run across my heart this year. . . ." He looks to his heart, in other words, for the thought that will get him going and get him to go on, to start on the new year of the life he has to live, still. Still alive, he needs to find the heart to go on, which is why he looks to it. This is a recovery to which I can relate.

His search takes form in writing, for writing, it seems, attunes Nietzsche to his heart. He sounds surprised when listening to the tune: a thought that "runs across my heart" is not the same thing as a thought one puts in one's mind in self-possessed thinking; it is more like being overcome by a thought that has come over you. Only after Nietzsche listens to that strange thought at the heart of him does he write the line whose content is so frequently analyzed, "Someday I wish to be only a Yes-sayer." That is his resolution for the new year, his resolution to begin again, recovery. It comes *to him—from his heart*, where thoughts that are not first his own touch down and others run across.

*The Gay Science* ends with him struggling to sustain this effort, for resolve is difficult to maintain over time and takes all the heart he finds. It is as if the heart it takes to write was given up in writing it; the heart possessed in writing, spent. No wonder the oscillations, the moodiness, the swings, the ups and downs, energy followed by exhaustion, high spirits by low, that run throughout Nietzsche writing. Having spent all he received from his stranger heart, he is by the final paragraphs of *The Gay Science* writing at odds with himself. Spirits are failing him as the new year goes on, dark thoughts coming over his heart as he recovers it, and a shadow cast upon the pages as he writes the book of his heart. "I slowly paint this gloomy question mark at the end" is how he puts it. And yet, in the gathering darkness of his gloom, he finds that "the spirits of my own book are attacking me, pull my own ears and call me back. 'We can no longer stand it,' they shout at me; 'away, away with this raven-black music. Are we not surrounded by bright morning? And by soft green grass and grounds, the kingdom of the dance? Has there ever been a better hour for gaiety?'" To which Nietzsche, cheered, responds and says to his heart, "Is that your pleasure, my impatient friends. Well then, who would not like to please you?" (§383). He takes heart and is cheered when his writing confronts him as a second person, "you," the spirits he now resolves to please. The hour for gaiety, good humor, and high spirits comes to him from these others he finds inside him at odds with what he has been identifying as himself.

Is that where we are given the heart to take when we take heart?

All this remains frustrating to many of the young people I meet in the classroom. Not only did Nietzsche not believe there were final answers to heartfelt questions of meaning and purpose, truth and wholeness; but, despite this, he still addressed his heart and the matters associated with finding and having it. This leaves him in an even worse position, they say, of listening to questions without having the belief that would access answers. Why would he listen to his heart or speak to it, they wonder, if it does not let him see clearly his purpose in life or tell him directly who he is? Others contend, by contrast, that he is not really listening to his heart at all, for if he did, he would not falter so frequently, not find himself lost so often, not be so divided and at odds with himself that the spirits of his own book have to cry out to him, and not be so beside himself that he has to utter heartfelt cries to his very heart to get up. The heart, they say, is where answers to these questions and questionable states are found. It is where I am who I am, they say, and if I find it, I can never lose myself.

But I don't find that heart to be one I call mine, is what I would like to tell them. Do you? It's hard to have a heart you call mine. Nietzsche knew that and tried not to live heartlessly. "Up with you now, come on, my old heart!"

Zarathustra's words had been on my mind for some time as part of this conversation with students, but they came to the forefront of my attention when they appeared as epigram to the final chapter of *With the World at Heart*, a book written by Thomas Carlson, my good friend. I read a draft Tom sent to me at the beginning of 2018, the year that some months later would find my heart laid bare and in the hands of the doctors and surgeons.

If you read Nietzsche *with the world at heart*, you know that "Up with you now, come on, my old heart" are words of cheer. They belong, Tom taught me, to a cheer that sustains the work of education—which is my work, the work of my students, and the shared work of learning that we transmit to each other across the generations that divide but also sustain us. In the humanities, where we are students and professors, the learning concerns the lessons of life, the most present one being the matter of a transition college students are making into the less sheltered world of grownups, becoming an adult or maturing, in other words, but this is of course only one of the many transitions that constitute the time of living life. A living life, made more of transitions than states, more of recoveries than arrivals, will become . . . and that means lifelong learning and recovery of the power of beginning. Being a teacher of life's students, Tom reminds me, means communicating to those students more than goals to attend to, more than power to perform such functions, more even than the skills, competencies, and information that is such power. It means communicating cheer with all the rest, for it is surely easy for youth of whatever age to lose heart standing on the edge of this or any next step in life—on the verge of commencing this new year in which they find themselves still alive, still writing the book of their heart. "Up with you now, come on, my old heart," a teacher wants to teach young people to say as they look for the heart they need to go on, growing older with the new year. But, Tom reminds me, and I need fewer and fewer reminders these days, "Up with you now, come on, my old heart" is also the maxim heard by the old, who, growing older with the new year and finding themselves they still live, experience the need to stay youthful. If young people must learn to become old, to age, old people must learn to stay young, to remain youthful so as to go on with life's transitions. Education in the lessons of life is about the lifelong learning of both from the other. It takes heart to go both directions: as if aging were sustained by remaining young at heart—and stops dead when the heart for youthfulness does, too. The aged teacher again stays young at heart when he, living on, learns to become a student adopting the maxim they teach him, "Up with you now, come on, my old heart." My students, the good ones, and my children, teach this cheer to me. The good old teacher I become when I learn from my students, the teacher who is a lifelong learner learning life's long lessons, confuses youth and age, aging and juvenescence, and in such confusion, enters and remains in perpetual recovery, back to beginning again.

It leads me to wonder: How old is Zarathustra, teacher of the Overman? The first sentence of the book tells us he is thirty, a midpoint of life, one of its turning points. Is this tale a record of youth growing old or age remaining young? It is difficult for me to tell which, as for me, too. Is it the case of a crusty old man looking to find the heart to stay young at heart? Or is it that of an exuberant youth finding the heart it takes to age? Either way, "Up with you now, come on, my old heart."

I am trying to cheer the students, too, then, when I dwell on Zarathustra's "Up with you now, come on, my old heart!" Many resist this communication. They do not want to learn it. They do not come to class looking to find heart. They come to class looking to solve problems and acquire problem-solving skills, even in classes in the humanities where I teach. Isn't that what thinking is about, they say? Isn't that why one takes a philosophy class, to learn problem-solving skills, skills for ordering one's thoughts in ways that transfer to any situation, by which we mean career or job, or at the very least skills that help you succeed on the LSAT? Supposing that thinking must be methodical to be critical and that critical means problem solving is why a lot of students think they should study philosophy, so when they come to read Nietzsche, they are rightly perplexed. This is not thinking, they say, or if it is, who needs it?

The students' suppositions are not lacking in support from many of us who teach in the humanities, and especially from our accrediting agencies. All are often desperate to promote the humanities classroom by claiming it is a place where one acquires transferable skills and competencies, not something soft and elusive like a heart. These are skills we believe belong to a mind that can perform well in corporate systems and teams. We tell students that employers want minds that have them. We might be right about what employers reward, we might not be, but regardless, I find it disheartening to hear that what an education in the humanities is *really* about is acquiring these kinds of skills. When we teach thinking reduced to a technical skill, we don't find our hearts giving us much to think about.

More and more students, too, are disappointed with their encounter with the works when read this way and leave the classroom dispirited . No wonder. They are right to be disheartened. Going back to Descartes, I can see why: such thinking is heartless from the beginning, and it supposes a thoughtless heart. How can they be expected to take heart from thinking without one? How can they be expected to find heart in a classroom where there are only skills and solutions to be found? There is no solution to the problem of the heart.

Nietzsche and his texts are especially good counters to this creep into my classroom, "Up with you now, come on, my old heart!" one of the best.

Zarathustra speaks this heartfelt cheer in the fourth and final part of *Thus Spoke Zarathustra* in the chapter titled "At Noon," another midpoint. It is, I remind students, the hour of what the desert fathers called the noonday demon, *acedia*, the sloth, listlessness, or indifference that overcomes me when the day's work is done but night has not yet come and the day still remains. Still alive, one is tired, but finds no place to rest—at noon, there are after all no shadows in which to hide—so one wanders constantly without arriving anywhere, or one stays still but is moving all the while: restless, in short, trembling. When one stops, it is not so much by putting oneself to rest as by being overcome by restlessness and collapsing, fainting away into sleep. Does a brain tremble and grow faint like that? The noonday demon, the shadow that falls over you at noon, when you find yourself still alive, is surely a matter of the heart.

This is what has overcome Zarathustra in that memorable moment when he commands his old heart "Up with you now, come on." As I continue with the students, I remind them that a shadow had come to haunt him in the previous chapter, "The Shadow." It follows him everywhere, crying out "Where is—my home? I ask and search and have searched for it, but I have not found it. O eternal everywhere, O eternal nowhere, O eternal—in vain." Zarathustra tries to outrun this shadow, but it is noon and there are no shadows in which to hide, no darkness in which he can take shelter from the one shadow that follows him every-where. The only shadow that remains when the others vanish is one's own. The strange shadow that does not go away when all shadows vanish in the lucidity of noon is yours. It is his shadow, then, I say to the students, and he finds he cannot escape it. Lis-tening to its cry, Zarathustra stops running, stops his perpetual motion, and identifies his shadow truly. He identifies *with* this stranger he hears and speaks to it, this strange thought of him-self that shadows him: "You have lost your goal. With this you have also lost your way." Overwhelmed, understandably, by the thought that shadows him: it is all in vain; I am entirely lost, no way, no goal, and therefore without direction, for there are no meaningful directions to take when everywhere is eternally everywhere else—understandably overwhelmed by the thoughts weighing on his heart, Zarathustra can do nothing more and col-lapses in sleep.

Healthy active minds, the students know, are buffered from thinking like this that the goal is lost, the purpose abandoned, and that there is no direction or guide. Vital engagement in one's projects and losing oneself in the flow of challenging and pro-ductive work with frequent benchmarks to check in on keep such thoughts away, the students have been told in popular literature offered by the experts, and if they don't read it, they have the campus clubs and other resources to tell them so. But when you can no longer put your heart in it, these bufferings lose their effectiveness and a shadow falls over our thoughts. When everywhere seems no different from everywhere else, everywhere is nowhere at all and arriving anywhere, no matter how lofty an achievement, always a disappointment—so what, now what? Today's healthy mind is immunized from such thoughts, but they might still cast their shadow over the heart. Anyone who has one would feel it and tremble, feel it tremble and shudder. Maybe even faint away, like Zarathustra, and sink into the repose of the ground, "the stillness and secrecy of the many-hued grass" (388).

Heartfelt is a hard way to be.

That stirring of the heart might be the wellspring from which came the hard thoughts that overcame Nietzsche—or so I tell the students—the thoughts that are so hard for any of us to think when they take possession of us, but which Nietzsche is famous for thinking.

In a cold and heartless world, it is easy for oneself too to grow disheartened, and nothing be done with cheer, neither work nor play. This mood can often prevail in our education of young people as we take on the role of preparing them for success or social advancement in a cold and heartless world. When "blindly raging industriousness, this typical virtue of an instrument" (GS, §21), is among the highest of virtues in a society where everybody is supposed to be an entrepreneur, we are simply too old to be young at heart and too young to have the heart to age.

This absence of cheer is evident in the Soothsayer Zarathustra meets. The Soothsayer's declaration of the vanity of it all ("All is the same, all in vain, nothing is worthwhile") expresses his realization of "blindly raging industriousness." It is as if in him the modern heart had heard what Nietzsche was telling it about itself and the industrious entrepreneur at last realized what it means to have the modern heart: "great weariness." This weariness is not the same as being exhausted from each of life's efforts nor is it the same as being exhausted from a hard day's work. Those have a luxury to them, and the exhaustion can be enjoyable. The "great weariness" is instead tired of endlessly participating in the endless back-and-forth of effort and exhaustion, the alternation of accomplishment and rest, tired, that is, of the Sisyphean labor of pushing the boulder of life up the hill day after day only to see it roll down the other side and need to be pushed up again. Recovering the strength to expend and expending it only to experience the need to recover the strength to expend again and again—that is what the great weariness proclaimed by the Soothsayer wants to drop out of. Dis-spirited, he has, I would say, lost heart, but he does not have the modern heart buffered against that loss. He collapses, can't go on, won't go on. . . .

The Soothsayer's weariness threatens to overcome Zarathustra, too, as he faints away into a deep slumber and soft grass at the thought of the eternal in vain that shadows him. I admit the temptation. But where the Soothsayer does not have a heart that feels its loss, the great weariness "stings [Zarathustra's] heart," is felt by it. A heart not a brain, a heart not a pump. The heart that is lost in great weariness is, paradoxically, the one that is found: the heart is found to be lost. Losing heart can be a telling loss if you listen to what the lost heart tells: lost, it tells that you have a heart to lose. You should respond to what it tells. Speak to that lost heart, then, your lost heart, that heart you listen to when you have lost heart. "Up with you now, come on, my old heart!"

This is what I would like to tell students.

Though the thought that shadows Zarathustra echoes the Soothsayer's declaration of the vanity of it all, the Soothsayer does not find that he has lost heart. Zarathustra does, praying it. The heart Zarathustra speaks to is found to be lost and failing. A lost heart is a difficult thing to find, a difficult disclosure of truth. The Soothsayer avoids it: though he talks *about* it, he does not address it, listen to it, or speak from it; he does not take it to heart. Zarathustra does.

Zarathustra listens to his heart frequently, more times than I had noticed on previous readings. It is not hard to get students to see this. When they do, they are likely to connect listening to your heart with having a purpose in life. Finding what's in your heart, they might say, means possessing an unshakeable, firm determination that pursues goals indefatigably (my word, not theirs). Zarathustra does indeed have a purpose, his fiery speeches evidence that, he is teacher of the Overman and learner of the lessons of eternal return. Teaching is his vocation. Listening to his heart may very well make for a purpose-driven life, then, as some of my students say, but if I am to agree, I must also say that that drive is enough to give him pause, a hesitancy that takes form as an address to the heart that is there to be taken up. "Up with you now, come on, my old heart" is spoken from the heart to the heart that hesitates before following the vocation of a heart it listens to and calls mine.

Most of the times Zarathustra listens to his heart are when some change has overcome him. Changes of his heart make up the plot of his life; they punctuate his book, each chapter of which begins or ends with him listening to one. The prologue even suggests that the book is the story of Zarathustra's changing heart and what happens when he listens to it. These are its opening lines: "When Zarathustra was thirty years old he left his home and the lake of his home and went into the mountains. Here he enjoyed his spirit and his solitude, and for ten years did not tire of it. But at last, a change came over his heart, and one morning he rose with the dawn, stepped before the sun, and spoke to it thus" (121). The story commences, the adventure begins, with this departure, casting-off in response to his listening to the murmuring of his changed heart.

What happens to him when he follows his heart? Those who have read the book know that it calls him to be a teacher, the teacher of the Overman and that means being one who thinks the abysmal thought of eternal return. Following that call, becoming an educator, means leaving the solitude of his refuge on the mountain. Descending to the valley, he loses himself among people, vitally engaged as he is in the heartfelt work of spreading the word, teaching. Time goes on, and he grows tired, tired from caring so much to teach others, few of whom listen and hear, and tired from spending so much of his spirit on caring for these others, few of whom are students and treat him more like consumers treat a merchant who does not have what they profess to want and hasten on to others who will give it to them. Feeling himself slipping away in the pity that draws him outside into the marketplaces, streets, and classrooms where they gather and his teaching fails, he withdraws, grows reticent and steps back to the solitude of his sheltered cave on the mountaintop—where he convalesces and there recovers . . .

. . . recovers the need that drives him to go down again. The second book begins again with him, still alive, addressing his heart in another of its changes. In fact, it begins almost exactly like the first: "Zarathustra returned again to the mountains and to the solitude of his cave and withdrew from men, waiting like a sower who has scattered his seed. But his soul grew full of impatience and desire for those whom he loved. . . . One

190    BOOK OF MY HEART

morning, he woke before the dawn, reflected long, lying on his bed, and at last spoke to his heart" (195). A change of heart will never be the last, it seems, bringing Zarathustra back to the point of needing to start again. Following his heart, Zarathustra inhabits a life with these highs and lows, peaks and valleys, up the mountain only to recover the need to go down the mountain, down the mountain only to find the need to go up the mountain, seemingly going nowhere at all. It's not hard to imagine one would grow tired. Not just tired of going up. That is exhausting and calls for going down. Not just tired of being down. That is exhausting too and calls for something that gets you up. But weary of the oscillation itself of life's transitional adventures, its adventurous transitions.

"The aim is lacking. 'Why?' finds no answer." (Nietzsche)

"I'll go on." (Samuel Beckett, *The Unnamable*)

"Up with you now, come on, my old heart!" (Zarathustra)

It is clear that when Zarathustra listens to his heart, he does not find answers to the nihilistic questions why, wherefore, to what end or what good is it. Some think it would be nice if he did. Many wish he would have an answer to the question why we should get on with the days of our lifetime, an answer that would give a purpose for it all; having one would justify the command to my old heart and give a reason for it to obey. Students are unsatisfied and disturbed that the imperative is without reason; it troubles them that it issues from an abyss, groundless, that it emerges almost spontaneously. This means, they see, that if listening to your heart means finding your purpose, which may very well be true, then that purpose is abysmal. Following your heart walking a path without ground.

The third chapter also begins again with him speaking to his heart at another turning point in his life story. He is leaving his

friends and students in the valley for the solitude of his mountain, again. "I am a wanderer and a mountain climber, he said
to his heart" (294). It is not easy, clearly, taking on the seemingly
endless ups and downs of living this existence disclosed in his
heart. One who finds the heart for it will doubtlessly bruise it.
"Thus Zarathustra spoke to himself as he was climbing, comforting his heart with hard maxims; for his heart was sore as
never before." Having heart, he will bruise his heart.

When convalescence means recovering the strength to fall
down again and again needing to convalesce, anyone with a heart
would hesitate. Put this way, it is easy to understand why living
a life listening to your heart and following its calling would be
full of hesitation and hesitations. Like Zarathustra's. The prologue to his book is in fact an extended delay of, a hesitation
before the moment when he begins, begins to "go under" with
the weight of the changing heart he has taken up. I can feel his
hesitancy in the unfolding of that prologue. Zarathustra "began
to go under" (122) at the end of the first numbered section, but
he is still beginning to go under ten sections later, fifteen pages
in my edition, at the end of what is still only prologue where the
line is repeated as the final one: "Thus Zarathustra began to go
under" (137). Students who read closely are confused, or else they
use it as evidence to claim Nietzsche is a bad writer. But the repetition of the line, the delay it spans, bespeaks the truth of listening to a heart you call mine and beginning the new chapter
of life it opens.

In the meantime of that delay, Zarathustra speaks to his heart
five times. It is as if he speaks his hesitation to his heart—and
it is as if his hesitation before taking on the story of his life
assumes form in speaking to his heart. These addresses to his
heart, these hesitations, are the form taken by someone who

assumes the being disclosed in his heart, what many would call their "purpose in life," their vocation. Nobody without a heart can live purposefully, and yet nobody with a heart can live purposefully without hesitating in that purpose. When Zarathustra listens to his heart, he hears it calling to him with a vocation that gives him pause. "Up with you now, come on, my old heart!" is spoken from the heart to the heart that hesitates before following the vocation of a heart it listens to and calls mine.

# II

# HAVING A HEART IS A CHRONIC CONDITION

*April 2019.*

*The problem of my heart solved when we asserted ourselves that day in the operating room and now with the pills and the chemicals, the question of my heart remains—its "nonsensical phrase" beating on returning again and again. I cannot not hear it and ask about the matter. What am I to do with my heart? It's a question, not a problem: it does not have a solution. A question I have to live with. A chronic condition. Having a heart is a chronic condition: so long as there is time I have one; so long as I have one, there is still time.*

*It is beginning to look as if the solution to the heart's problems doesn't make the question of having one go away.*

*I am having a hard time accepting a cure for the heart that means being cured of the heart. I want to be able to say "Having a heart is not a problem" with a positive tone, but knowing that problems have solutions, I also know that not being a problem can be worse. If "having a heart is not a problem" means having a heart is a question, a chronic condition, it is difficult to say affirmatively, difficult to leap into unreservedly, difficult to do in a heartfelt way. A chronic condition is hard that way: you have to say "yes" to it if you want to be so as to say "no" (or "yes") to anything at all.*

# 6

## THE HEART'S IMPERATIVE

As I look to the future to which I was opened by aortic valve replacement (AVR), having a heart appears to be a chronic condition. To be a student of life's lesson now, as my friend Tom Carlson might put it, is to learn to inhabit that condition, and that means learning to speak to what I hear when I listen to my heart and to listen to what I hear when I speak to it. That's what good students do: more than know things, they speak and listen in response, listen and speak in response.

Where do I look for teachers? Teachers, not just experts who have knowledge and information that let us know the pump at the heart of the bodily machine well enough to repair it, but teachers: those from whom I might also learn and take heart. Friends and family, of course, people who have called or written to me, visited and lived with me still. They above all, they first of all, but also other others. Notably those I find on the shelves in my library, as I pull books that have been there for many years: Nietzsche and Augustine, they have proven heartening; also a handful of artists, mostly modern and contemporary visual or performance artists whose work attracts me, draws me on and moves me, for reasons I am trying to understand here. Their books are open on my desk or else on my lap a lot these days as I sit in the warm air on the porch, hanging out into the hollow where we have settled, listening to the song of birds fill the emptiness and watching the brilliance of light dangle in the filaments of the trees. . . . Tehching Hsieh, Yves Klein, Bas Jan Ader, Christian Boltanski. A selection of literary artists, too, mostly fiction, some criticism but literary in style: Karl Ove Knausgaard (*My Struggle*, but also his writings about art); Henry David Thoreau (*Walden, or Life in the Woods*); Cormac McCarthy (*The Road*); Maylis de Kerangal (*The Heart*).

It's an odd collection, idiosyncratic, perhaps hearkening back to the days of the personal library before everything was available to everybody everywhere with access all the time. A personal library from times before we all consumed all the same cultural works—those that appear at the top of our Google search or on the lists of what the publishers and production companies sell to us. Few colleagues who look at those names would see them belonging together, except in me. Friends and family, too, think it odd but for other reasons: many of those works are dark and despairing, they say, you should be reading something happier, something that will put a smile on your face, they tell me.

But I can't live without these teachers these days. I don't live without them. They are what gives the heart it takes, the heart I need, to get on with the one I have.

It is time to make a day of it. I have been too disheartened for too long now, and the days have "sloughed past uncounted and uncalendared," as Cormac McCarthy puts it. Dealing with the matter of my heart, I can't avoid the question that Stanley Cavell said was the challenge Thoreau's *Walden* poses to us: "How to earn and spend our most wakeful hours is the task of *Walden* as a whole . . . what writing Walden is."

I had been reading and writing with much seriousness about Thoreau before my defecting heart made it too difficult to go on, but he comes back now. The entirety of his time at Walden Pond was an experiment in finding the heart for making his days, a hearty effort at a lifetime and its days. He in fact uses the phrase "make a day of it" at least twice in *Walden*. Once when he is speaking about hoeing his beanfield, he says "I sometimes made a day of it" after he shares the ominous thought that "the night-hawk circled overhead in the sunny afternoon," as if he saw the end in night already in the beautiful sunny day. And once before in the more programmatic chapter, "Where I lived and what I lived for," when he writes: "Let us spend one day as deliberately as Nature, and not be thrown off track by every nutshell and mosquito's wing that falls on the rails. Let us rise early and fast, or break fast, gently and without perturbation; let company come and let company go, let the bells ring and the children cry,— determined to make a day of it."[1] His daymaking belongs to a kind of resolve or determination, not a resolution on this or that in particular (I will quit smoking; I will be nice to my brother; I will do my German homework for an hour every day) but a resoluteness that welcomes a day's arrival by letting what comes come, and go, as it is. Whatever it is, Thoreau tells us, "Let's make a day of it" by letting it come and letting it go. When it is a matter of making a day of it, not making success in this or that specific task or project, determination means letting, letting be that lets go, letting go so as to let be. He lets the day be as a way to make one.

My admiration for Thoreau's text was equal only to my incomprehension of the character. It wasn't that I couldn't understand what he said. I could make some sense of that, creatively if I needed to, and when I couldn't, I had the benefit of more than a century's worth of experts who had written lengthy books or pithy essays illuminating the writings themselves and the contexts, social, political, economic, scientific, and so on, in which they were embedded. What I couldn't understand was the teacher: him, the character, his person, the way of being in the world, most especially the vitality to which he testified, the cheer he seemed to radiate, especially in his best-known book *Walden, or Life in the Woods.* How could he be like that? As I look back now at the broken strands of what I had been writing about then, I am tempted to put what confounded me in terms of his heart: Everything he did at the pond, and he did almost everything that belongs to our daily life, he did wholeheartedly. In all that he did, he put his heart into it. What could have given him all the heart it took for all that he did? Where did he find it?

One of the motifs around which my perplexity was organized was dawn. The enthusiasm with which Thoreau appears to greet the day, to welcome the dawn knowing full well that the day that had dawned included a night, a nighthawk that already showed itself in the middle of a sunny afternoon, that the day would fade in twilight and disappear in the night, like the mournful sounds he listens to when he first arrives in the neighborhood of the pond: cows lowing in the distance, whippoorwills chanting vespers, and the doleful hoot of the owls, "like mourning women their ancient u-lu-lu."[2] But still, "let's make a day of it." It didn't seem to matter what he did with his day, what plan or program he devised for daymaking, what was on the to-do list and how much of it got checked off, he always seemed to make a day of it, each day, whatever it was. Some of the things Thoreau did with his day seem silly or a waste of time, some outright excruciating, more the stuff of a painful, miserable day than a successful day. He hoed seven miles of beans all day in his field and still claims to have made a day of it. He spent a day on his belly on the ice of the frozen pond peering into its watery depths just to make a map of its bottom, and that was a day that turned out

well. He watched red ants battle black ants through a magnify-
ing lens without missing the day. How boring, I would say;
hardly what you would call making a day of it; but his heart was
in it, in everything it seemed, and that could make a day of it, of
anything—even a walk through the cemetery of fallen leaves that
the face of the earth had become for his own recovered soul, as
he said in the beautiful essay "Autumn Tints."

I might be able to understand him, but even then, can I, too,
find the heart for it?

When your heart fails, a dark light shines on the experience of
time and our chronic condition. What I saw in that light
sometimes made it look like what you see in pictures of a book
that is often with me these days.

The book shows Tehching Hsieh in a "one year performance
piece" called *Time Clock Piece* (April 11, 1980–April 11, 1981) during which he punched a time clock every hour on the hour, each
day, every day, for a year. A chronic condition if ever there was
one! That's all he would do, attend to his chronic condition—by
punching the time clock. It didn't take much strength, and it
didn't take much skill, anybody could do it. What did it take?

Heart?

I first encountered Tehching Hsieh when a friend gave me his
book *Out of Now: The Lifeworks of Tehching Hsieh*. That was several years ago, while we were visiting his farm in Wisconsin, well
before we were attending carefully to the matters of my heart. I
was intrigued but went back to other projects that absorbed me
more, other work that seemed more fulfilling, writing about
Thoreau, for instance. I did not feel the need in which possession of the book mattered, so it sat safely stored, closed, on a
shelf. These days, however, I spend a lot of my time with it open
on my desk or lap, reading and looking at the pictures in it. I am
trying to figure out why.

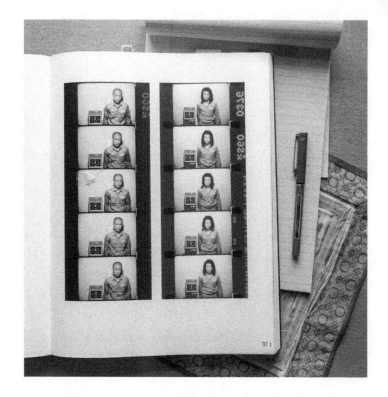

In *Time Clock Piece*, Hsieh reduced the days of his life to time itself and the chronic condition it imposes. Punching a clock every hour on the hour was his way of saying "yes," "present," "here I am!" to that chronic condition. It is hard to imagine what would move him to do it or what could give him the strength to go there so frequently. He must have heard some strange imperative from beyond reason, common sense, or any other thought that could be related to others.

An imperative of the heart?

An alarm clock sounded the call. With each appearance before the time clock, a still image was taken on a reel of high-8 film, making for 8,760 pictures. When the year was over, Hsieh

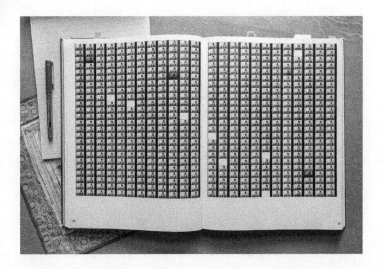

screened the film reel in its entirety at a performance scheduled for April 11, 1981, at 6:00 p.m. Showing what? As Adrian Heathfield sees it, Hsieh "becomes a sentient witness of time."[3] A witness of time, not an observer who has looked at it from a safe distance and can tell us all about it, but a witness of time in the sense of one who testifies to it in a person and body shaped by the experience of suffering it. A witness who is also evidence, then—evidence in the flesh. A witness who is also victim, someone who got so close it touched him and he was burned. The book on my desk shows it.

Time, in that series of images, the chronic condition of human being. Hsieh is made to be what he is by it appearing in him. Even more so, I imagine, when the images are moving in a film reel. Aging run fast forward—and it runs in only one direction, unrelentingly and frighteningly down. That's the chronic condition he inhabits.

Quite a few viewers would call it unhealthy. If that is where a heart takes you when you listen to its imperative, many would say it is crazy to follow it. Hsieh does look a bit like a madman, or a derelict, at least a drop out. That is more or less what he did: drop out of our everyday days. And he did it for more than just one year. The year before *Time Clock Piece* (1980–1981) Hsieh performed *Cage Piece* (1978–1979), in which for one year, he sealed himself in his studio, in solitary confinement, inside a cell of iron bars measuring 11′6″ × 9′ × 8′. A friend cared for him, bringing meals to him and removing a waste pail for him, but there were no distractions, nothing to entertain or occupy him, nothing to pass the time in what I have to imagine was a lot of time that would *not* pass. Each moment might pass—in fact, that might be all they did, for none was in any way at his disposition—but time always remained, returning eternally the same. He had time (nothing but time) yet could not do anything with it (time but nothing).

He must have sunk into a profound boredom. I did, and I had been doing it for only a few months. There was almost nothing to do but time. Imprisoned in a cage, Hsieh was indeed "doing time" (the title of his contribution to the Venice Biennale of 2017), only to find, I have discovered, that time is not something one does; in such a state of destitution, there is nothing one can do to make it pass any slower or faster; it is something (nothing) one suffers. Chronic condition.

One year after leaving the cage, he performed *Time Clock Piece*, then, after *Time Clock Piece*, three more one-year performances, each beginning a year after the previous one ended: *Outdoor Piece* (1981–1982), in which he did not enter any indoor space for an entire year; *Rope Piece* (1983–1984), in which he was bound by an eight-foot rope tied to artist Linda Montano all day every day for a year; and *No Art Piece* (1985–1986), in which he, an artist, did not make art for a year. Eight years of a lifetime delivered over to the work of an art that drops out of the days in which we live meaningfully with others together with things that belong to the projects that make up our worlds. *Rope Piece* makes that

experience of deprivation painfully evident as being bound to
Montano by a rope meant it was difficult for the time he spent
with her to be spent in any meaningful way. There she was, but
not as a meaningful part of his days. There all the things of his
everyday days were, but tied up as he was, they did not belong
to projects that could pass the time. Taken all together, Hsieh's
one-year performances make for eight years of this. "Let's make
a day of it" takes on a new urgency from such destitution. Chronic
condition.

I was not living anything like a day those days when my failing
or convalescing heart gave me over to its chronic condition. I was
not greeting my days, their dawn was not something I crowed
about, nor was their twilight an end I celebrated having reached.
Hsieh, too, does not look like he is crowing about the day ahead,
but he does seem to rise up, stand tall, shaggy and drawn but tall,
and say "Yes," punching the time clock, saying "Here I am!" to
the chronic condition of his days.

   When I was forced to drop out of everyday life, Hsieh's resolute affirmation of that condition proved illuminating—it shined
a light, a dark light to be sure, not just on my present state there
but on the lost everyday. My friend Tom Carlson once wrote
words that come to mind now: "In light of that darkness," Tom
writes, "they confront the barest, essential condition of worldly
life and its possibility—conditions now illuminated by their very
darkness."[4] The darkness can be illuminating, Tom reminds me,
illuminating of the very conditions that make for the everyday
days we usually inhabit. That is not the same as saying that there
is a light to be found in the darkness, or that if you pass into the
darkness you will pass through it to the light. That would be
reassuring. Saying instead that the darkness is illuminating, that
a dark light shines there, is a harder teaching because calling to
a harder place to learn one's lessons. For it to be the case, for the

darkness gathering around us to be illuminating, one must attend to it, dwell in it and on it, and that is not easy in cases of our chronic conditions. Whence perhaps my fascination with Hsieh's work, *Time Clock Piece* especially: What is to be seen in the dark light of this apocalypse of the days? What lessons are learned by going into our chronic condition with him, or anyone sick and ill, for that matter?

"The times are out of joint." In these days when I am trying to recover the heart I cannot not listen to, it is hard, hard to "make a day of it," as they say, much less put together two good ones in a row. The days are hard to start (it is tough to get out of bed in the morning), sad to end (difficult to say good night and anticipate the last), and tough to get through in the middle when my defecting heart grows faint (the noonday demon or Zarathustra's shadow is always lurking and an afternoon nap ever tempting). It might start out well, but as Peter Handke puts it in his own "Essay on the Successful Day," "in the middle of the enjoyable afternoon, fear of the rest of the day."[5] Even if I should succeed in making a day of it and the day turn out well, there remains the night, the night that belongs to every day we make. Every day I make collapses into this, its night, and I have to do it again. What dawns on me when I greet the day is the ending of the day and the end of the day is having to face its dawn again. It is relentless, the days and the need to make one, then another one, and another one, and so on. No wonder there might be "fear of the rest of the day" in the middle afternoon. The noonday demon is very real. Where is the heart, one wonders, for what I remember Stanley Cavell calling "the willing repetition of the days," the willingness to take up each day everyday repeatedly, chronically?[6]

"The times are out of joint." The hours don't add up to a day, much less weeks or months. Indeed. I don't know when I am.

The clock is no measure that is mine, the calendar no map on which I find myself. I don't find myself scheduled like the others in my family or my workplace, my name does not appear on the lists with theirs. The here where I am is not found there where they are. My time is not theirs, theirs not mine. I am not involved with the things they have and have to do. It feels strange not to see my name on the daily schedule on the calendar at home where the names of everybody close to me are written. They all have things to do, people to see, and places to go. Me, none.

I would like to be able to seize the day, but it doesn't seem within reach. I sleep a lot but never much at once, so I am awake a lot—even at night when I should be sleeping so that I can be awake during the day when I sleep a lot. It's confusing. The times are all mixed up. I can't tell if I should sleep more or less, be more awake or more asleep. I wake mostly to sleep, even if I get up with others in the house as they get ready for the day they have ahead of them. When their day begins to get busy, I go back to the night's business of sleeping.

"Seize the day" doesn't seem like the right maxim for me. It is good advice in general, but for someone who is not me in particular, and I exist always, *though not only*, in particular. For me, already too late for the day and behind the times, seizing it is out of the question. The very idea of seizing the day seems like "saying to a bootless man that he should lift himself up by his own bootstraps," as Martin Luther King Jr. once said. What I'd really like is to have a day, just to make a day of it, this mess, whatever it turns out to be, but my heart, my defector heart has left me without one. If "seize the day" is good advice, its effectiveness must be reduced to another instance by the question: "do you have the heart for it?"

I am tempted to call *Time Clock Piece* a one-year performance of submitting to that question. It didn't take much strength, and it didn't take much skill, anybody could do it. All it took was heart. For one year, Hsieh listened to the imperative of the heart and said "Yes," "Here I am" to the chronic condition of our everyday days. Is that the lesson to be learned in light of the darkness into which he descended?

*The alarm clock sounds the apocalypse of his days.* It interrupts the day, ruins it by suspending the differences that would make each and every one, blurring them in the indistinct fog of indifferent hours. What is made by listening to its alarming call is not a day but a barrage of hours at best, a series of drips like drops accumulating in a pile that is not gathered into an interrelated whole. Time, yes, but not collected into the days of our day-to-day life. Time, yes, but in the drone of its regular drip, nothing like the tempo of the living time of our daily life, which goes faster and slower from time to time depending on whatever it is that absorbs us and whether we are absorbed in it. In short, time utterly lacking the rhythm, pleasant or not, that makes for our days.

Ironically, *Time Clock Piece* called Hsieh into unclocked time and space. Ordinarily the clock measures out a day that belongs to the time that composes a lifetime, one moreover shared with others. Ordinarily, the clock makes for a schedule that organizes the day of everyday life and does so in common, binding us together in shared times. But nobody heard the clock Hsieh did, nobody else answered its call. It scheduled the life of nobody but him. It called to and for his heart, the heart he called mine. Responding to its call tore him away, dis- or ab-stracted him, from the life together with others that is one of the great advantages of passing the time immersed in our days. Deprived of its everyday functions, the clock sounds only the alarming call of time.

In such times, what sort of expectations could he have had? What could he expect—of the world, of his day? Very little if anything at all. He didn't even have a day, just a pile of hours. Without a day, he had nothing to expect, and without expecting, he could make no day to have.

In such times, what sort of memories could he have made? What could he remember when he had no rest from the barrage of ever more alarming moments without a moment's pause when he could recollect them? What even was there to remember when little to nothing could happen in times so brief and fleeting? His was hardly a life in which he could hope to make memories, and not making memories is not a lifetime, much less having the time of your life.

What could he expect to remember? What could he remember to expect? Only the moment of punching the clock. There is no future in that since the next moment is only another one of the same, nor is there any past since no moment ever goes away when it is the same always. Time, void and voided of all—the memories and expectations, memory and expectation—that fills them in our everyday days.

Without expecting or remembering, Hsieh could not engage in the activities that belong to the days of living time. He could not commit to anything, for he lacked the time to realize it, and he couldn't commit to anyone, for the time there was was not had in any way that could be given to or shared with anyone. He might have had all the time in the world, but the time was not available to him. Hsieh puts it bluntly: "In one hour, I could not do very much." There being nothing he could do, he had nothing to do; there being nothing to do, he could do nothing.

*He could not work*—certainly not productively, for how much can one get done in a series of moments that last barely a short hour, that only accumulate without amounting to anything? Starting most projects is senseless, meaningless, when the alarming call of the time clock will interrupt them in an hour. Ending most projects similarly meaningless, impossible, when the alarming interruption comes before they have reached fruition or been completed.

*He could not rest either*, for the recurrent sounding of the alarm put him back to work as the servant of time. All the trappings of the laborer—the uniform, the punch clock, the surveillance camera—only highlight this and its opposite: if he is meant to be a worker, he is an unemployed worker, a day laborer maybe put out of work by his labor in the service of time. Perhaps that is really the garb of a prisoner he wears? A prisoner of time, confined to a chronic condition?

*He could not dream*: "My dreams were always interrupted," he tells us (330). Imagine that, not even being able to dream! His most intimately intimate thoughts, his dreams, for himself and for others, broken apart, his interiority never able to collect itself because of the alarming call of his chronic condition.

*He could not be with others.* The talk that binds us to others fell silent and senseless to him. "Even if I were talking to someone, I would be thinking, 'I have to go and punch the clock'" (334). Attentive as he is to the time clock, he appears distracted to others. Talking with them, Hsieh could not focus on the exchange of words in which the world appears in common. He lived isolated from the others with whom he still found himself—with nothing to tell anybody or himself about how he spent his time because he didn't spend any time on anything. "What did you do today?" Nothing to say in response. How can you be with others when you can't respond to that most mundane and everyday of questions?

*He could not move freely.* How far can you go when you have to return to punch the clock every hour? His day shrank, therefore. Space was constricted and his movements confined, too, by the interruption of time.

*He had no things to do.* His to-do list must have been very small if not entirely empty, his calendar blank, unscheduled. About the only thing that could be on it was "Punch the clock," "Do time," chronic condition.

When "do time" is on the to-do list, it can become the only thing that is on the list, and that looks scary: a chronic condition. It's so scary that usually and for the most part, I try to forget it and live happily oblivious, never putting it on my list of things to do, instead filling and over-filling that list with more specific, more determined tasks. "Doing time" or "making a day" did not have to appear on that list, and I would forget all about it—at least that is how it was until an alarming call became the apocalypse of my every day, and I couldn't avoid the truth of their chronic condition: my aortic valve broke, my days shattered, and I was reduced to the dark point where "time" was about all I, too, could "do."

My to-do list shrank. In general I am not exceedingly busy or overscheduled, so that list is never overly long, but when my heart was failing, items were not getting lined out. After a while, it became clear that "live," "do-time," and, most important, "have a heart" had to be put on it. Once those were on the list, it became equally clear that anything else I did, which wasn't very much, could only be done according to my chronic condition. What was done was what my heart gave me to do, and moreover it was done in the mode granted by my heart. That is the sense in which having a heart is a condition. My condition last August and November, for instance, was such that "fixing the fence" was not a possibility I could call mine, maybe "cook the dinner" was, "help with homework" was probably possible, but "chop fire-wood" was a long way off. Moreover, just how I was when I cooked the dinner or helped with the homework was shaped by my chronic condition, sometimes more vigorously, sometimes more cheerfully, but oftentimes I just couldn't find the heart for it and did it lifelessly, listlessly, utterly lacking in spirit. That's what it means that you have to put your heart in it. I know because I could not. Is that what we see in the dark light of a broken heart?

Is that the lesson Hsieh learned? To listen to the heart's imperative and learn to do time? Marina Abramović, the renowned performance artist, tells a brief anecdote suggesting as much. Visiting him once after his one-year performances were over, she says that she "asked him what he was doing, he simply replied: 'I am doing life'" (352). In the darkness of eight years of one-year performances, Hsieh learned to do life, to do time. Is that all? What good is that? Why learn to put on the to-do list what you cannot put on the list and destroys it when it has to appear there?

In the dark light of my own failure of a heart, I feel as if I have come to the point where I can address that question—hesitantly, to be sure, but still respond: Because otherwise the list is a list of what to do with a life you don't live, days in which you aren't. Hsieh's story tells me as much. It is as if he had to have the heart to do nothing in order to go there where the heart to put into anything might be found. Hsieh's effort then is the effort to "do" what makes it possible to be in the doing of all the other things on that list, "to do life," as he said to Abramović, in other words, to make life into something lived, rather than something without living being in it. Even though "do time, "do life," doesn't usually appear on the list of things-to-do, it is nevertheless the unwritten, unstated affirmation underlying them all.

Sitting here with this book on my lap, I see what Hsieh called "doing life" as the work of the heart. He looks neither excited about it nor despondent. He has reduced his life to the acceptance of what must be accepted for anything at all to be on the list that constitutes the days of our days. He puts his heart into it, whatever it will be.

Hsieh inhabits a chronic condition not unlike that of someone who cannot not listen to their heart. Claire Méjean, for instance.

Claire is a character in Maylis de Kerangal's novel *Réparer les vivants* (in its American translation, *The Heart*).[7] Claire lacks the heart to seize the day. Indeed, she lacks the heart it takes just to have a day. Hers is failing, like mine, a chronic condition, not a crisis like a heart attack, but unlike mine, hers can't experience recovery. She needs a transplant. A myocardial infection, a virus that infected the muscle of her heart, has undone her. Fever, aches, and tiredness, "a sort of general exhaustion," eventually fainting, collapsing in shock on the streets of Paris, characterize life with her defector heart. She will soon die of it.

Needing the heart of another, "all she does is sleep." The day passes her by, like every other one. Sleeping through them all, each day is simply unavailable to her, perhaps because more fundamentally and essentially, she is not available to them. The heart it takes for that is failing her. The possibilities of a meaningful life in the world with others are still there: shopping with friends; editorial work at the office; lunch dates with her children—they all call on her at different times, offer her work or to take her out, but she cannot respond affirmatively, say "yes" or accept. She cannot find herself in those possibilities, and we never find her actually living out any of the ones that call to her. In fact, she can barely leave her room where she is imprisoned in the here and now. She is one of "those who are waiting . . . whose lives are restricted, suspended by the condition of a particular organ in their body," the heart. It's a terrible sort of waiting, a waiting "with no conception of the future" occupying a present with no expectation that the moments to come will bring

new times to remember or other places. It's a kind of deep boredom. A waiting that remains after the end has already come, as
if dead already. Dead time.

Confined to what is by her failed heart, Claire haunts an
apartment in Paris. She has relocated there so that she can be
close to the hospital, which now dominates and consumes the
space of her life. Her doctors don't want her to go very far in case
she collapses and, more hopefully, in case a transplant becomes
available. The place is hateful to her. She "feels an immediate
loathing for [it]." Her heart is still in her provincial home while
her life is here in Paris. The provinces are a place where she is
welcome. Paris and her apartment are not so welcoming, an
experience of rejection repeated each day when she is greeted by
the stairs that await her at the entrance. In fact, there is no greeting at all, only heartrending separation. "Climbing the stairs
gives her pain, each movement making her feel as if her heart is
separating from the rest of her body." Home, the place where one
hopes to put one's heart, is no home at all. The place where she
finds herself feels less expansive, more and more restricted and
restricting. The things that ordinarily provide ready access to a
wider world of belonging, such as the stairs that would let her
out and in, become mere objects achingly present opposite her.
She cannot use them without losing heart. "Day after day, the
space seems to close in around her, limiting and reducing her
gestures, restricting her movements, narrowing her entire world."

The space of the apartment is not all that collapses around her,
so too does time. Claire finds that "time seems to disintegrate
into a bleak continuity. . . . The alternation of day and night soon
loses its distinction, and all she does is sleep." Such sleep is deadly.
We should sleep to wake to new days. If we don't, our sleep is
death's. In the deadtime of this "bleak continuity," the days all
run together, leaving an immense "it" where there might be

distinct days separated by nights. We call "it" *time*, I think. "It" is hardly the time of a day or the time of a living human life.

When her defective heart is so far gone that she faints frequently, absenting herself from the life that remains without it, Claire's world becomes one without options. "She has no choice," de Kerangal tells us; she has to live in a bleak apartment near the hospital. "This is what it means to be sick, she thinks—not having a choice. Her heart has left her no choice." Claire has no choice but to be in this apartment in Paris where she never would have chosen to be, but she does not have the heart for being there and cannot say "yes, here I am" to what she has no choice but to choose.

Claire's case is worse than mine, but I can see myself in it. When my heart was failing and weak, my world grew similarly small in possibilities. The only possibilities I could see for myself were ones that already were actual actualities. It was difficult, in other words, to do what I wasn't already doing, which wasn't much. With few expectations, I inhabited a world poor in future. Most everything seemed impossible, especially to start—the day first and above all, and I would rise from bed only to cross the room to the club chair where I would sit for an hour or more before going downstairs. The possibilities that remain, the few that are there for me—sitting in front of the television, eating some toast, talking for a little while on the telephone, for instance—do not seem like possibilities anymore, for they are the only thing I can do. Having been left without options by a failing heart, the world that remains is hardly one we, Claire and I, can say we chose. But we have no other choice. We have no choice.

It's tempting to give up.

Tehching Hsieh did not give up. Though destitute of days, he kept punching time's clock, rising up again and again as if he heard in that drone, in "it," some imperative to go on and said "Yes, here I am" in response, "present," to time.

The artist statement that opens *Time Clock Piece* expresses Hsieh's quixotic resolve: "I, SAM HSIEH, plan to do a one year performance piece. / I shall punch a Time Clock in my studio every hour on the hour for one year. / I shall immediately leave my Time Clock room, each time after I punch the Time Clock. / The performance shall begin on April 11, 1980 at 7 p.m. and continue until April 11, 1981 at 6 p.m." The statement is dated April 1980 and signed "Sam Hsieh."

There was nothing binding him to do it, nothing and nobody compelling or forcing him to show up when summoned by the alarm—other than his word, and he meant what he said, which might be harder and higher than saying what you mean. There were also no external obstacles, forces blocking him from doing it. With nothing binding him to it, and nothing stopping him from doing it, the work is all about effort, internal effort. Nothing is hard about it, except wanting to. Hsieh says as much: an "inner struggle," he says, is the only matter at issue in performances done in situations of destitution like this; "what is determinant is the will," he says, and the "inner struggle" that the will is (324). *Time Clock Piece* lays it bare.

I have come to think of Hsieh's "will that is determinant," his "inner struggle," as rooted in the heart. If all that is needed is to want to do it, you have to be willing, and willingness comes from the heart. It is tempting to say that it takes a lot of will-power or self-discipline for Hsieh to keep his appointment with the time clock all those times. I would agree. But where does that come from? Where does the will find the power? What activates it? That's the mystery. It must come from somewhere other than itself, for he doesn't always have it, he has it sometimes but not always or forever: the record shows that he oversleeps from time to time and is occasionally late to punch the clock, sometimes but rarely even fails to show up at all. What he calls "the will that is determinant" must get its determination from somewhere besides itself, somewhere where its power of command falls short. I would call that "heart." The will needs—to find the heart for it. I know it's not advisable to correct an author when interpreting his work, but I wish Hsieh would have said "what is determinant is the heart."

His is remarkably large. Dedicated to arriving on time to punch time's clock on the hour, "Here I am," every hour, for a year, his heart has to be. He is not bursting with enthusiasm, and his look is anything but gleeful, but there he is, ready, punctual, present for it.

Most of the time. Sometimes he slacks off. Who wouldn't? Anybody with a heart would grow tired and miss a few hours. Anybody with a heart would chafe inside the constantly worn uniform and skip work once in a while. There are gaps, voids, in the stream of photos, and the punch card shows the occasional :01 or :02, sometimes even :04, where he was late and missed the hour, :00. There is a printed breakdown. The book I have on my desk in front of me shows both the lacunae and the misses.

He missed 133 times out of 8,760. That is about 1.5 percent of the time. His resolve seems good. I would like to be present to that much of the time of my day-to-day life.

Most of his misses came because he was sleeping (94). For many of the others, he was just late. The misses begin to grow more frequent in August (13) and peak in November and December (18 and 25, respectively). Having started the project in April, Hsieh probably grew tired as the year wore on. After the initial enthusiasm of a wholehearted beginning, it always becomes more

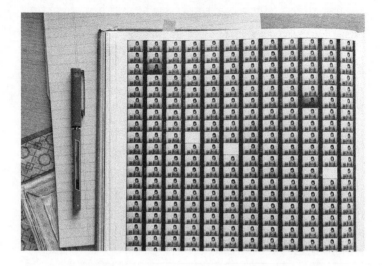

difficult to find the heart for whatever it is as time wears on—
on the heart that keeps us open to time, resolutely open to the
time that wears down our resolve.

By January, the misses are back down to seven, and in March,
the last month before the show came to an end, they are at eight,
with an anomalous sixteen in February.

With no cause or reason to be there, each and every one of the
times opened by his quixotic resolve offers a moment when he
could turn away from the time clock, ignore its alarming call and
do something more advantageous and absorbing, more comfortable and fulfilling—or else throw in the towel entirely, quitting
time and the chronic condition. However determined he was,
then, his heart threw him into time in which every moment was
an occasion for quitting as much as renewing the resolve that
opened him to the call of the clock. Hsieh is no quitter, however,
and he is not an escape artist. His art does not ask me to admire
the skills or pastimes of an escapist, be it escape from ties,

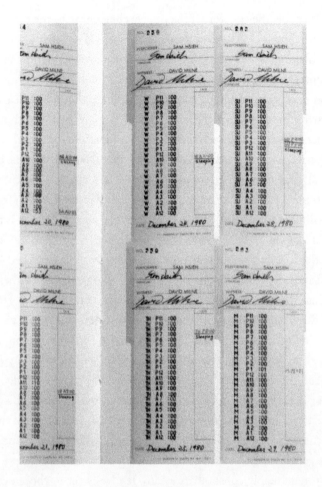

confinement, summons, or anything else. I find instead that I am asked to wonder at and about an unsettling resolve to stay, to stay with it, to stay in it, time and our chronic condition. The heart for that resolve to stay shows itself in *Time Clock Piece* in the mode of frequently coming back. As I see it, then, his quixotic resolution was a commitment to re-resolving, to a resoluteness that would resolve again and again resolving all resolve, frequently, in fact every hour on the hour. It takes a lot of heart.

Isn't this the case for all the projects belonging to the days of my life, though? All of my projects, the ordinary, everyday ones, art-making as well as a diet, a job or a marriage, gardening and keeping house, all take root and unfold in a chronic condition that implies re-resolving each moment. I see that quite clearly now in the dark light of Hsieh's art. We might prefer to think otherwise, approaching our projects, our identities even, and our experiences as if a resolution made just once would determine us for all time to come. But to think of projects, identities, and commitments as requiring only a once and for all resolution is in fact to think of them unconditioned by their chronicity—which is to think of them as ideas without existing in time or therefore world, idle entertainments of angels. The truth is, disclosed in the apocalypse of Hsieh's days, the resolution it takes for them being in time is re-resolving, each day every day.

Resolutely staying with it by frequently coming back to it calls for and takes heart, takes the very heart it calls for having. *It takes heart, so soon enough all your heart will be taken by it.* Spending the heart you have on whatever it is and all you do in your days, you will soon be spent. That's what it's like to be in the days conditioned by time. I can see it in the dark light of the witness Hsieh becomes. It's not obviously visible in one single image, one single time of the times. His gaze is steady, his expression remarkably constant. A steady resolve is set in those eyes and that jaw. The fatigue comes, of course, with time, when you put the images into a sequence and experience the relentlessness of it, the unrelenting barrage of the times to which his hearty resolve exposes him. Time wears on him and wears him down. It might not appear if there were not a sequence. If I consider each hour on its own, he looks set. Not particularly happy but not particularly sad, not angry about keeping his appointment with time and yet not gleeful about it either, just set and steadily so. It's not exactly determination, for he doesn't look focused on anything—"ready" might be a good word, though not eager. And yet, the series that puts together each of these steady moments of clear resolve or readiness shows the ravaging wreaked by their barrage. I can't identify one in particular, one of the times that would be singled out as the eventful moment when his devastation began or the ravaging overtook him, and yet it did. Steady and set, ready and resolute, in each and every one of the times, Hsieh is ravaged in all of them. Each is steady, yes, but all ravages—hair grows shaggy and unkempt; his back stoops and slouches; the uniform crumples and wrinkles; and he slows, is late, or misses some appointments. Voids interrupt the stream. They grow more frequent toward the end. When you gather together all the steady times and set them moving in time, as Hsieh does in the film that consummates the performance, you see it all fall apart. The steady gaze of his strong heart exposes him to that. It holds him open to the rundown, the breakdown, and the absence that ravages him.

He inhabits a chronic condition.

I do not feel prompt and ready, as Hsieh appears to me to be; much less am I greeting my days joyfully like Thoreau. What comes to mind more frequently when I think to describe my condition is a line from Cormac McCarthy's novel *The Road*, "the days sloughed past uncounted and uncalendared."[8]

The line comes up in a class I teach called "Heidegger and Being in the World." I added the title to the schedule of readings because of what I learned about it from a book (and an academic article) written by my friend Tom Carlson, *With the World at Heart: Studies in the Secular Today*.[9] McCarthy's novel describes a cold, heartless world, or rather a postapocalyptic ruin in which the absence of world threatens at every moment. The world is cold without sun as ash and climactic leveling have left all in a shroud of grey. Cannibals roam the devastation of a now heartless world. Nothing changes, students rightly point out, everything the father and son fight off, most frequently the cannibals, returns to be fought again, and they reach the shore only to find it disappointingly the same as the land. There is only a "bleak continuity" of time and space. Seasons don't pass or even come, and the father wonders "What time of year? What age the child?" Indeed, in the cold and gray, amidst the destitution of time and world, "the days sloughed by uncounted and uncalendared."

At home, mine did, too. There were no cannibals. I was in fact taken care of by others, friends, doctors, and so on, who did it all for me, including leaving food on the doorstep and bringing meals upstairs to me morning and night. Relieved of all my obligations and commitments to others, there was nothing for me to expect to remember, and similarly deprived of work by my weak and failing heart, there was nothing for me to remember to expect.

The uncounted, uncalendared days taken care of by others are free, unattached, with nothing to do. "Each providential to itself," is a phrase McCarthy uses earlier in the book. It sometimes seems like bliss. No to-do lists. "No lists of things to be done," McCarthy writes. "The day providential to itself. The hour. There is no later. This is later."[10] "Live for the moment" becomes a real option when "later" makes no sense. Providential only to itself, the day reduced to hours without a future is uncalendared, leaving it free, entirely free, open and unscheduled. "Be here now" (Ram Dass) becomes a maxim one can realize. It might be a dream come true, heaven on earth, true happiness, bliss. An inexplicable providence may have been smiling on me.

Such thoughts did not escape me in my own sloughing day. I dwelled in a certain leisure, and I dwelled on lots of matters. I read in Peter Handke the wondering remark: "Bring about a successful day by pure dwelling? To dwell, to sit, to look up, to excel in uselessness."[11] I did a lot of sitting, a lot of looking, and it made for a lot of dwelling, just dwelling. It was excellent uselessness. A friend even said the best writing I had ever done grew out of it.

Yes, the unnumbered days are free, and with nothing to do because nothing I can do, they provide for a certain leisure and bliss. The "sick role" and the hospital are tempting.

But one might want a little more. One might want something more than happiness and bliss. One might want to live in the days of a lifetime. That is what I was coming to see in light of the darkness gathered around me. I learned to long for a to-do list, McCarthy's "list of things to be done," the list that much of the time I hate and want to be free of. Such lists always seemed to me to represent everything we do without our heart being in it, everything contrary to the logic of the heart, but illuminated by the darkness of my lost and failing heart, the to-do list appeared differently: brilliant in that dark light, very much desired, now that I could see the truth disclosed that there will come a time, like this one, when I have none.

In the absence of days, a to-do list doesn't make sense. "Do it," when? "Do it," before what time? "Do it," in conjunction with what else, who else, for whom? All those questions that make the to-do list meaningful make no sense when "there is no later" and the days "slough by uncounted and uncalendared." Having the list gathers all those around it. I want to be involved with all-involved. I must want the list that comes from and calls forth those involvements. I long to see my name on the calendar, along with the others, my projects scheduled around theirs, on the clock, I need to be on the clock, as it were. I want a clock and a calendar, and for that, I need there to be some numbering to the days, so that they can be countable, by others, too, and then maybe count. Where can those numbers come from?

"My days are numbered." I wrote that once. A frightening sentence, a hard one to pass on yourself, but I wrote it in August 2018, when I was taking account of the expiration dates soon to be inscribed on my heart, specifically on the valves of my repaired heart. You can read it in the first chapter of this book. "My days are numbered." When I listen to my heart, that's what I say in response. Still. Even today, after it has been repaired.

Writing that sentence again now is frightening, but I can see its generosity. It makes for a turnaround, a rebound that throws me back into the days of an everyday lifetime, clocks and calendars, schedules, to-do lists and all. "My days are numbered." The expiration dates that numbered my days make them countable: by numbering them, they can count—relieving me of days each providential to itself and opening the possibility of a later, a calendar, days interrelated in memory and expectation. Illuminated by the darkness of my failure of a heart, I see that the good life may very well be lived with the heartfelt awareness "my days are numbered," for the numbering that marks the days might be the condition of making them count, too.

"My days are numbered." It is not despair talking. It comes from the heart.

"Out of now," the title of the book of Hsieh's lifeworks, is another way to say it: "out of now"; the end is near; apocalypse; my days are numbered. The numbers in the book on my desk tell me as much.

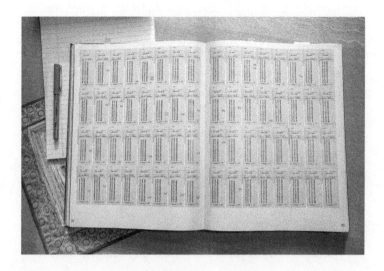

But is there a rebound here, too, in Hsieh's descent into the chronic condition? Is Hsieh's punching the time clock every hour each hour perhaps the source of it counting?

Tim Etchells, a renowned artist of durational performances like Hsieh, thinks so. Reporting on what he felt when he attended the film where Hsieh presented the work, Etchells writes, "I was silenced by what I saw. I think I was frightened" (355). It is without a doubt scary to be so close to someone whose inner life and deepest thoughts are so remote, so far away consumed by the chronic condition that has consumed his life and left only a void before us. We have no idea what runs through his mind, what he is thinking in that chronic condition, such that he has fallen into an unimaginable solitude, or rather into a solitude that can only be imagined, painfully so, maybe maddeningly, by us. Etchells admits being horrified by someone so disciplined about descending into this devastation of the days, this nothingness to which Hsieh reduced the world. He is not the only one. I, too, was horrified at seeing someone so intent on manifesting an emptiness I suspect might lie at the heart of my own days.

And yet, in the resolve that voids the world, reducing it to a frightful darkness and emptiness, a chronic condition, Etchells also sees its significance given back. There just might be a rebound that comes when we look into what the darkness illuminates. To this end, he tells the following story in the form of a letter to Hsieh. The events he narrates happened at a festival where Hsieh is showing photographs taken from *Time Clock Piece*. It is shortly after the one-year performance was over.

> "This is day 53," you said. "This is day 54. This is from day 55." [The session begins to run late.] It was over-running. But you seemed not to care, or not to notice. "This is day 212," you said, "and this is day 213." Once you'd shown one it seemed important to show the next. Each day matters, after all. And each hour, and each minute matters, too, each of them in their sequence and their uniqueness. There is not one more important than the other. (355–56)

Hsieh is counting the days, marking them, even if each seems unremarkable, with a number, just day 53 or 54, a mark that does nothing more than note them happening without saying anything about what happened or did not happen. There is a noticeable flatness to the gaze that numbers them and the tone that reports them, and yet there is also an obvious earnestness to recording each moment: counting them counts, for they count. Hsieh has exacted this counting of himself. The heart's imperative? Counting each and all. The hours, the minutes, they counted, so much so that even as time is running out for recollecting the memories he made—Hsieh will soon be "out of now," the hour scheduled for the presentation over—even as his allotted time has come to an end, he is not phased, goes on, without regard for the clock, telling their unremarkable story. In fact, the days count more than the space allowed by the everyday clock allows him to say, and when the days, hours, minutes of his chronic condition count so much, there is a lot to count, so, recounting it to others, Hsieh runs late, overruns. The unremarkable story is so important that it exceeds the end and will make everybody late for whatever else it is they have to do. He has been given more time by attending so carefully to his chronic condition of being in time.

Is this what it looks like to have made a day of it? Accepting the heart's imperative, does he have time now and can make a day of it?

Don't we all want more time? I certainly want to run a little late on life, keep going after the end of my assigned times, like Hsieh at the festival. Punching the clock every hour on the hour, saying "yes" to the experience of the chronic condition, was Hsieh's way to find time. He found a lot of it, more than the schedulers of the festival gave him. The work he did in *Time Clock Piece*, doing time, was therefore anything but killing time. Doing nothing to kill the time, he had a lot of it.

It didn't take much strength, it didn't take much skill, what it takes is heart.

Things are beginning to turn around.

So, too, with Claire Méjean. The darkness of her days shines a light on what keeps them open: an imperative to be available, ready—the heart's imperative. It calls to her.

One night, in the midst of the "bleak continuity" of a life lingering in "the unending darkness of the place" where "the alternation of day and night has lost all distinction," she receives a surprising call, a call about a heart that has been found. It turns out that pursuing this heart is a lost cause, it is "too small and poorly vascularized" and has to be refused, but following the call of that heart, things and the time in which they happen are different for Claire. "After that, the nature of time changes—it regains its shape. Or rather takes the shape of waiting: hollow and stretched out." This is a new kind of waiting, unlike the bored waiting of sleepless nights and wakeless days in which there is no future in any of her tomorrows. This new waiting is an almost inspired waiting, not boredom but anticipation. She waits for a future she cannot give herself: she waits on the heart she can call mine. "From that point on, the only purpose of the hours is to be available during them, knowing that the transplant operation could suddenly become reality, a heart might appear at any moment: I must stay alive, I must be ready." She is listening to an imperative ("I must stay alive, I must be ready") that comes from the heart she has found to be lost, the imperative of the lost heart she has found lost. Her attentiveness to that imperative means making herself available to the hours that remain. Life matters. It is imperative to be present to *it*, so that I will be ready for the heart that will come when it will. Waiting, having nothing but time is not boring, the time had urgent. "I must stay alive, I must be ready." When she listens to her lost heart, there is a future in her tomorrow.

And with that, clock and calendar return. "I must stay alive, I must be ready. Minutes become supple, seconds ductile, and finally fall arrives." The "bleak continuity" of "it" becomes the units of a day with stretched out, ductile, moments of minutes and seconds in which there is time for something that can turn out one way or another, supple. The seasons return, one passes into the past and the next one arrives from the future. The present differs, in other words. Tomorrow has a future in it. "Fall arrives," the alternations that make for the rhythms of our days return. In that time, Claire can begin to be at home. Her apartment in Paris begins to resemble a place where the days of an everyday lifetime might be had. She "resolves to bring her books and lamps to this tiny apartment. Her youngest son installs wifi for her, and she buys an office chair, a wooden table, gathers together a few objects: she wants to start translating again. / Her editor is delighted by this news, and sends her Charlotte Brontë's first publication. . . . Each day spent working yields a slender batch of pages." No longer suffocating under "the power of now" but in a present in time, she has something to do, her work, a modest mission but a meaningful project. Her editor would agree. He is involved in it with her. Working a little, sharing the work with her editor, Claire is back into a minimum of everyday life.[12]

And with me? Are things beginning to turn around for me?

*"The alarm clock sounds the apocalypse of his days."* I wrote that to describe the devastation of days reduced to a chronic condition. But "apocalypse," the theologians remind me, does not mean just the end of days. "Apocalypse" also means, in fact means literally, "unveiling," lifting the veil, and so could also be rendered as "disclosure" or "revelation," truth laid bare. That's what is seen in light of the darkening of the days, their truth. Hsieh exacts that truth. His days having come to an end, what remained was the uneventful goings-on and ongoing uneventfulness of time remaining to pass and passing to return. This was the situation into which I too had been led by the heart I called mine. I was confined to the barest minimum of involvements—in work, with others, with the daily tasks of keeping up the house, and so on. Like Claire Méjean.

The truth is we will one day be delivered over to this condition. Aging will get us. All hearts will grow weak. They all will fail. And if they don't, if we come to an end before ours ends, we probably wish it were not so. I know I do. I live with the hope that I will grow old enough for my heart to fail again, for I don't want to die young or early.

Could this be the beginning of my rebound? Is this my saying "Yes" to the chronic condition of having a heart I call mine?

In my case, wanting to have more time, this hope for the future, in fact means hoping for repeated heart failure. The artificial valve inside me bears an expiration date, and when it expires, my heart will fail again and they will repair my failed heart, I hope, with another artificial valve that, I hope, will also expire some time before I hope I do, and so on and so on. Until they can't. I want to live on, I want more time—which means I want to live with this failure of a heart. In fact, I hope to live long enough that it does again.

In both Claire Méjean and Tehching Hsieh I see the future that belongs to the time I have. So, too, in my sloughing days. My heart failure will return. I will be back here one day, and it will be worse. I see it now, already, the truth to come laid bare, apocalyptically disclosed, the end of days. This is my future, how it will be. No more to-do lists. Just lists. A catalog of things I look at, hopefully admire; maybe an inventory of projects people do, but not me. There will be no "to-do" on my lists because my failing heart, like Claire Méjean's, will mean I am powerless to do, anything on the list that remains in the time remaining.

When I look today at Tehching Hsieh in his chronic condition, I don't see just another. I don't look at him and say, "thank God it's not me." Claire Méjean, too. When I read the story of her heart failure, I am not reading about just another. I don't look at her and say, "she is just a character in a novel, and anyway her case is not mine." I read and look today with my heart in it, and putting my heart into it, I see in each of them the future that belongs to the days I have to live with my heart.

Should I read this way? Should anyone? Many of my academic colleagues caution against it. They tell us to read or look more critically and stick to writing about what we can and do know about the works at issue. It's hard these days for me to do that, though, read and write, look and write, without putting my heart in it. What comes from that, then, comes from the heart.

# 7

## PUT YOUR HEART IN IT

*May 2019.*

*Heart surgery was a leap of sorts. I didn't so much put myself into the hands of others as throw myself into them, the hands of people who were mostly strangers. That leap gave me a future, one that now opens in the days before me, a lifetime that yawns much wider now than it did in August 2018.*

*The move that I thought of then as a leap into surgery was, I see now, a leap that leaped through it (in several senses of "through") into ordinary days and everyday life. This means landing again in the world of to-do lists that only grow longer the more I line items off them, the world of schedules that need to be arranged then kept so that multiple and diverse lives can be coordinated and managed, the world of frustration with things that break or that won't do the job I need them to do when I need them to do it, the demanding world of being with others who want things of me as much as they want things for me, and so on. It was different during the seemingly timeless now out of time just before and after surgery. Life was straightforward then. There were not a lot of things that cluttered my day: wake when they tell me to; eat the meals they bring me; walk down the hall and back a couple times a day, eventually to the mailboxes at the side of the road; write until I could not any longer; and sleep, a lot. Most of it was already decided, there were few decisions to make, and others cared for me.*

*Coming back, however, homecoming and homemaking, means
I am landing again in the zigzagging paths of days and days made
of diversions and dead-end frustrations but of course also of achievements, mostly small but even so, and of delights: everyday life lived
alongside ordinary things, together with people and tasks to do. I have
a future, and that means making plans and preparations, hoping and
dreaming, for myself and the others for whom I care. If I used to think
of heart surgery as something like a leap into a void without certainty
of outcome, I can see now that the success of the surgery was probably
more certain than the everyday days it will have given me in the times
ahead.*

I often think of my heart surgery in terms of what the religiously
musical might call a "leap of faith." The theologian or philosopher most often associated with that phrase is Søren Kierkegaard. Even though he never uses the phrase "leap of faith,"
Kierkegaard does speak of a leap, and he does speak of it in a
discussion of faith. What is less often remarked is that his discussion of leaping and its relation to faith occurs in the context of
considering passionate movements, what I am tempted to call
heartfelt movements or, on a good day, hearty ones.

What Kierkegaard means when he thinks about faith in the
context of leaping and about leaping in the context of faith should
be distinguished from what some of the religious as well as some
of the antireligious frequently take it to mean. On both sides
there are those who think we can leap because we believe, that
it makes our leaping confident of its outcome. We might believe
theologically—for instance, believe in a higher being that looks
out for us such that we can be confident it will all turn out all
right for us; or believe in a higher power operative in all events
such that everything that happens, whatever it might be, happens for the best. We might also believe in less traditionally

theological ways but ones that still retain a shadow of religious belief—for instance: believe the cosmos itself is the best of all possible worlds, including in its optimization a place for me; or believe that the universe is arranged with our, and even my, good in mind, that the universe cares about me and my good. We might also believe in ways that seem to discard theology and its cosmological shadow entirely—for instance: believe in ourselves (the doctors or myself) and our abilities to provide for ourselves, collectively or individually. Any of these beliefs, the story goes, precede the leap and make it possible: they give confidence, ultimately security, and without that security, nobody in their right mind would leap.

None of that is what Kierkegaard means by leaping when he talks about faith or by faith when he talks about leaping. What such believers (and their critics) call faith is used instead to eliminate the situation in which leaping is called for, Kierkegaard would say. Those leaps are not really leaps. By assuring us in advance that all is well, that whatever happens happens for the best, this so-called faith lets us know that there is no need for fear and trembling as we advance through the world, that the days harbor no possibilities other than those that are known already to be actually good, or, put differently, that the days will present no actualities other than those good possibilities we already know constitute it. One does not leap into such days so much as walk easily into them. A leap implies a void or an abyss, at the very least some hurdle, an obstacle.

The leap about which Kierkegaard speaks is also not a way to throw ourselves into believing something even though we have no method for getting our thoughts there. The leap of faith, in other words, is not a way to go from not-knowing into knowing, from unbelief into belief. On Kierkegaard's telling, leaping is instead how we move when we don't know what to believe yet go on without the guarantees of belief assuring us it will work out. Honestly, it's absurd. Which Kierkegaard admits, saying famously that faith moves "by virtue of the absurd," not with good reason. When leaping means moving by virtue of the absurd, the faith involved cannot be the same as having good reasons to be sure that it will all be for the best and you will come out of it well. This can be one way to distinguish faith and belief.[1]

The absurd basis of the leap is connected to Kierkegaard's insistence that faith is a passionate movement. The importance of such movements is discovered in those situations, more common than we imagine, he says, when we need to go on but find that knowledge and methodical thought, do not move us. If we move, go on nevertheless, such action is sustained by something more than reasons, preceded by something more than deliberation or calculation. It is passionate, Kierkegaard says. Passion doesn't need to know or be sure of the outcome to move; it moves before it knows all or even adequately about what it is getting into and what is drawing it on. We are moved—passionately, by passions, even when we ourselves are no longer able to move ourselves deliberately. This is why passionate movements are risky, why passion does not forget but supposes anxiety, and why many moral philosophers hold them in low esteem.

Religious faith, Kierkegaard holds, is exemplary of passionate movements and bold leaps in that it has before it, object of its aim, a by-definition incomprehensible or paradox. This incomprehensible or paradox confronts the individual with whatever it might be that necessarily confounds reason and then asks that individual to become someone who takes it to be true. Kierkegaard, rooted in European theological traditions, gives as example the incarnation, the God-Man or miracle proposed by Christianity. For an individual to become the one where that truth exists as true, Kierkegaard says, faith must do what there is no good reason to do—namely, take it to be true, and that means being, actually becoming, the believer in whom its truth is true. With no good reason to become the believer, the passionate movement of faith thereby is and does what cannot be explained or justified, its very existence is groundless, its coming to be whatever it is based in the absurd. It leaps, in other words, and that leap into existence, making real the paradox that there is no good reason to believe, is what Kierkegaard calls the highest of passions, the most passionate of passions. In short, faith's coming into existence, becoming the individual who believes, is passionate—it's also absurd.

Perhaps then faith's leaping is not really a movement of thought or mind at all. Maybe it is the heart that leaps faithfully—even if all of them are defectors and will defect.

When we confronted the problem of my failing heart, we did a fair amount of research, quick research to be sure, but there was time, time to come to know what we were moving into. We read about it, we talked to people in the field, we did our best to know the background and credentials of our surgical team, we talked to colleagues who had gone through it before, families who had dealt with the recovery, and so on. In short, we did all we could in advance with the time still available to us to ensure that our deliberations took all the evidence into consideration so we could be confident that we had good reason to be making the moves we would decide to make. We tried to be methodical in solving the problem of what to do. And what all these calculations gave us to see was that a functioning heart would come out of the surgery. Anybody who knows or listens to those who know would conclude the same thing: the likelihood of repairing a heart by aortic valve replacement (AVR) is very high these days, especially if you control for someone my age, my overall health, and support networks, social, financial, and otherwise. This made us reasonably confident that surgery was the solution to our problem and that things would turn out well.

But, when time was up and the moment came, when we were on the verge of moving into the future our methodical deliberations had given us to see, I hesitated. I was afraid, and I shook. Despite knowing it would turn out for the best, I didn't move naturally or easily into the next step of the plan. If I moved, which I did, a lot, I moved without going anywhere—that is to say, I trembled. In place but not at rest, restless. All the knowledge we had gained, all the reasons we had for moving forward confidently, still didn't make it easy to actually do it, to actually do what we had decided to do. That remained a leap, and I trembled as I stood on the edge. I still wept as I left the house the night before, leaving Oscar and Claire, my children, with their grandmother while Stephanie, my wife, and I went to Charlottesville to spend the night closer to the hospital. Knowing things would work out for us, I still felt cold, cold fear, as I was taken away by the surgical team that wheeled me down the hall to the operating room that morning exactly one year ago today. I still shook as I spoke whatever it is I spoke about with the anesthesiologist whose face is the last thing I saw before I was overcome by the drugs that caused me to fall into a deep sleep before the potassium cardioplegiac used in lethal injections stopped my heart.

My leap sounds more like a fall. Agent or patient? Clearly a patient supine on the table. Perhaps it wasn't something I did, then, as they moved me, down the hall and off into that deep sleep?

While it seems as if the passionate leaping of faith is reserved for extraordinary actions such as becoming a believer or a heart surgery patient, in fact, Kierkegaard points out, those leaps are only exemplary forms of a leap that is more involved in our existence and actions than we might imagine. It takes passion to be, he says, and landing in everyday life is a leap of faith.

Kierkegaard saw quite well that reflection and methodical deliberation may very well assure us of an everyday course of action, tell us the right way to live our life, and even offer pleasurable ideas of an entertaining existence. But he also saw that the ideas constructed by all our serious and deliberate reflection offer no guarantee of actualizing, making real, the certainties we know or see in this kind of thinking. You can't think yourself into coming to be something, even when you know it is the right thing to be. A leap is required to cross the gap. It takes heart, I would say, to cross that gap. A mind alone doesn't do it.

We believe otherwise, Kierkegaard says. We believe that we can think ourselves methodically into being this or that and doing this or that, but this is to forget the transition from thinking to being, to forget that we have to become the being we conceive and become it in the everyday days of our chronic condition. Maybe we can in certain simple matters requiring little feel for existence. Coming to be someone in whom some mathematical truths exist as true, for instance, is not so hard for me: I can easily make myself be the believer of $2 + 2 = 4$. But in the weighty cases of existence, ones where I take up the burden of having my heart, this falls short: it was a struggle to make myself be the I who does aortic valve replacement surgery, even though I am the I who knows the numbers are in his favor. I know there is a great certainty of success, but am I also that certainty that I know? Often not.

Cases like this, matters of my heart, Kierkegaard insists, are in fact more like the everyday realities we inhabit. Most of everyday life is not as easy as being one in whom the certainty

2 + 2 = 4 exists. In matters of everyday concern, methodical thinking surely does belong to the project of completing the to-do list, but it really only brings me to the point where the list is written and a plan is made. Problem solved on paper or in my head, there remains the question of its existence, and that means me becoming the being who makes the solution exist. I have written the list, I have solved the problem of deciding what to do, but the way forward, into existence, the way to make myself be it, do it, anything whatsoever, can only be a leap—over the edge. That leap is the passion it takes to be, the heart I must put into it. Action of the simplest, most mundane sort, ordinary everyday being, even getting out of bed in the morning, eating lunch in the afternoon, and coming home in the evening, takes passion, always, he says. You have to put your heart into it. Heartless thinking does not enter into ordinary everyday being, practical daily life.

After five nights at the hospital, homecoming: I returned, was welcomed by friends and family. I was coming back to everyday life, and that should be occasion for joy, the joy that accompanies every great return and recovery, especially a homecoming, but I still struggled to find the heart for the days to which I had returned. I spent a lot of time in a recliner chair that friends who cared had arranged for me. I sat or lay there, watching, out the window at fading light and falling leaves or at images on the television screen, all passing without my holding onto them or caring about them or much of anything. There was only a world without myself in it on one side, screened images and objects observed, and me on the other, pushed back in the chair.

From where I sat, it wasn't hard to see the activities of everyday life and the others involved in them: getting kids from school and taking them to soccer or guitar; teaching a class; eating dinner with my wife; even cutting grass. I could imagine what it would be like to do all those activities, but I could not see myself doing them, they were not mine. There was a list, as it were, but it was not a list to-do and it was not assigned to me, my name was not on it.

Yet another way to say this is that driving, mowing, teaching, and so on were possibilities I knew very well, but I could not find myself in those possibilities and thereby make them actual possibilities actually for me, ones I called mine. They belonged to a kind of imagining captive to itself, giving itself ideas very productively but ideas that presented only images. "I guess that is possible," I would say. Knowing well that those things, people and tasks make up the meaningful activities of a day, I could, in other words, picture the possibilities of a significant life, but I just couldn't see myself in the picture, actually in it.

I could not claim the day as an urgency mine for the doing. I didn't have the heart for it. I wouldn't leap in.

That is perhaps why I was struck so powerfully one morning by a particular picture, the artist Yves Klein seeming to leap with all the heart I could not find. The picture is called *Leap Into the Void* (1960).

It takes a lot of heart to leap into the void, I thought to myself. Klein makes it look easy. It also looks exhilarating. A man in space defying gravity, as if the weight of matter had been lifted and he were rising, ascending to ever-new heights, elevating endlessly. The "pure bliss on his face" testifies to the joyful experience of this gravity-defying leap.[2]

The image of Klein's leap originally appeared in a special issue of a journal, a newspaper, Klein himself published, just once, titled *Le journal d'un seul jour* (The newspaper of just one day). It bore the headline "Yves Klein presents Sunday, November 27,

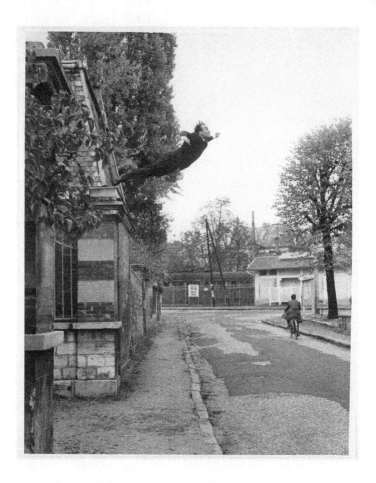

1960." Talk about making a day of it! He claims it as his to present. Leaping into it appears to be a way to seize the day and having seized it, say it is mine.

It was April 2019 when I came across the picture of Klein leaping, about six months into my homecoming. I found it in Adrian Heathfield's account of Tehching Hsieh's lifeworks, *Out of Now*. I had seen the picture before but not thought much about it until now when it seemed as if it were telling me something must change in my life. "You have to throw yourself into things," it seemed to say to me. "Seize the day," it commanded. I had to admit that was good advice. Perhaps that is what I found so fascinating about the image: the enthusiasm of an apparently whole-hearted leap. Was this picture to be a source of inspiration? Could I take heart from it?

The gravity defying feat of such a leap comes about, Klein imagined, through the dematerialization of art. When we "make art immaterial," he says, we can "levitate to another dimension."[3] That dimension belonged to a utopia to which Klein believed art could lead humanity. He sometimes described it as a new Garden of Eden. Composed of an immaterial art, Klein's Garden of Eden would be void of the matter that calls for care in our less-Edenic gardens, and without matter or care being called for, there would be no to-do lists, no urgencies of the day, no call, in other words, for all the planning in which that care takes form and no need, either, for the effort and hard work that realizes the plan. Freedom! Bliss!

The meaning of materiality for Klein was shaped by the mid-twentieth century, postwar society being fashioned at the time. Characterized by the explosive growth of consumer culture, commodity capitalism, and the technological domination of nature, this society is easily characterized as materialistic and one for which materiality means lots of material things being manufactured. Klein's leap into the void, taking place in 1960, amidst that materialism, makes sense to me as a way of transcending the mess. The materialism of all the consumer products, fashionable commodities, and plastic to which such materialism attaches us still make for a messy life, one cluttered by ugliness and burdens that bind us. I sympathize with Klein's art of dematerialization as a leap beyond it. What we imagine makes for our affluence ties us down and messes up our lives.

Klein's leap into the void thus bears a spiritual significance. It is a struggle with materialism and the distortion of the human spirit that it works. By disregarding objects and the production of objects (canvases, sculptures, and so on), Klein's art was a dematerialized performance that exulted in pure spiritual freedom—his leap a sort of jump for joy, a jump with joy, an exhilarating performance. The spirituality of his leap is expressed in a speech Klein gave in Dusseldorf in 1959 where he dreams that "we will all become aerial men, we will know the upward force of attraction toward space, toward nothing and everything at once: earthly gravity having been overcome, we will literally levitate in a total physical and spiritual freedom." Negating the gravity of things means, for Klein, attaining a highpoint of the human spirit. The driving force of this upward ascent is dematerialization: negating material matters removes all that weighs us down and we rise. Our spirit is then free, he declares, free from ties that bind us to grave matters of the earth (gravity) and free from matters, material matters, that limit the spirit. Realizing the spiritual ideal of dematerialization, he continued, is the work of art. This is suggested in the phrase "the dematerialization *of* art," where the genitive is ambiguous, both what art does and what art is. It makes a void in which pure spirit is found, limitless and free. In fact, then, the void is for Klein a spiritual plenitude, and the seemingly negative movement of dematerialization a positive step toward spiritual fullness. This means *Leap Into the Void* is really a leap into the fullness of the human spirit, a leap into a utopia free from weighty matters and the spirit of gravity.

No wonder he looks so gleeful. Dematerialization has its utility. When reality is immaterial and the matter of things no longer concerns us, levity triumphs, it's easy to leave the earth behind, and it's easy to be assertive, seize the day. It's not hard to make light of things of no matter.

Calling himself a "painter of space" and claiming his first work was to sign his name on the other side of the sky, Klein claimed to "regularly practice dynamic levitation."[4] One "must be capable of levitation," as he says, if one is to reach the position from which one can sign that signature on the sky. Leaping and floating thus become interchangeable for "aerial men" in the fullness of the void. The dematerialization *of* art assured this unearthly capability. It makes things of no matter, realizing a fully spiritual performance.

There is a glorious sort of insouciance to this leap: the look on Klein's face registers the mood, utter bliss unconcerned by any prospect of falling. Inconsiderate of where he might land, he appears not to care about what will come next, where he is going, what the future holds.

I see the attractiveness of the insouciance. I feel the draw of endlessly high-spirits. My friend Emmanuel Falque, too. He wrote a book, *Métamorphose de la finitude*, in which he portrayed insouciance as a certain high point of existence as a Christian believer. Christianity's highest symbol, the resurrection, signifies for Emmanuel just this: " *'transformation' du souci* [care] *en in-souciance* [insouciance, carefree living]." Believing-being lives "sans souci," without care, "insouciantly," he says, because what it has it has like the birds of the air in the parable— because they are provided for, not because they take care to reap or sow. Be then "without worry for your life" (Mt. 6:25), the gospel says, or as one could also translate Emmanuel's translation, "live without care for your life." What Emmanuel calls *"le 'sans souci' de la providence"* does not stem from the fact that the Christian has something different than others. Rather, it concerns how the

Christian has whatever he has, and how he has it is joyfully because at each moment how he has it is by having received it, moreover received from the Holy Spirit.[5]

Living like "the birds of the air" with what I might call Emmanuel's providential insouciance, confident it is cared for, or like Klein's "aerial men" who leap for joy with a look of insouciant bliss, is surely tempting. I, too, may have written some pages somewhere, maybe regarding Thoreau, in which I come close to promoting something that might be construed as insouciance as the mood or disposition of a secular happiness. But these days my heart won't let me leave it at that, and I listen to the thoughts that come from it. Insouciant and high-spirited is certainly not how I left the house the night we listened to my heart and followed it to the hospital, nor is it how I was when I was taken into the operating room, nor how I find myself now in the days when my heart is very much at the center of my thoughts precisely because I can't seem to find it. Listening to my heart, I can't leap like Klein. His leap looks inconsiderate of the heart where I find reality to be very material. The glorious insouciance of Klein's leap now looks despairing, as if it says you leap without fear of landing when it doesn't matter.

That's *not* how it looks when you leap with all your heart. I was wrong when I said that, and I find little to take heart from in Klein's *Leap Into the Void*.

Some people, I know, have had the good fortune of having their leaps turn into recollections that look like Klein's. They are blessed, or just lucky, to remember leaping as such. When leaping into the days becomes a memory like this, one has lived happily and it becomes easier to tell the world that this is what passionate leaping, putting your heart into it, looks like. But one says this having forgotten that it is how the leap looks in the recollections of someone who has landed safely already. I don't want to begrudge the happy their happiness; it is a terrible thing to resent the happiness of others, to assume, as I sometimes do, that the appearance of happiness belongs only to idiocy or the deluded. But people should be careful about portraying the leap, passion, and following your heart from the time and place of someone for whom the outcome has already been decided, and moreover decided that it turns out well. That time and place is one of recollection not anticipation, the time and place of looking back not looking forward—a point of view that easily forgets about the heart that is put at stake in such leaping, the heart that stands on the edge, on the brink, the moment it leaps ahead. In that moment, the one I call mine hesitates, stutters, needs goading and encouragement. Maybe Klein did come to the edge and hesitate, maybe he did need to pray "up with you now, come on, old heart," but he does not let us see that. He appears to leap in possession of a heart that never fails, and that, I would say, is no heart at all, certainly not one I could call *mine*.

One could also leap like a couple other artists, ones whose willingness not to will against gravity and its spirit made the leap into a work of falling. I am thinking first of Tehching Hsieh in *Jump Piece* (1973), another work I found in Adrian Heathfield's book.

*Jump Piece* is more mundane than Klein's spectacular *Leap Into the Void*. Hsieh jumped from the second-floor window of his house in Taiwan, recording the event on a Super 8 video camera. What happened is exactly what you would expect when gravity rules. He landed, crash-landed, really, on the earth, breaking both his ankles.

.

.

.

The unlimited freedom to fly might be an entertaining thought and image, but the facts, like gravity, bring us down to earth. Flights of fancy that rise eternally might satisfy a wish for transcendence, but we have to face the fact, as Hsieh did, of gravity and the grave matters of life on earth bound by it.

Some will surely say that this is self-harm and willed suffering. In fact, some did say that. Hsieh himself is reported to have said later in his career that he considered the work "immature, an unfortunate harbinger of future self-destructive pieces."[6] But you could also think of it as a matter of the heart faced with the facts of gravity and the weight of being earthbound. Stupid? Maybe. But it takes a lot of heart to leap knowing you will fall and land but not knowing how. How will you land? The logic of the heart that leaps without an answer to that question looks very foolish to a heartless thinking, but when you are bound to the earth, your heart feels a tug, the spirit of gravity, that leads you into the grave matter of being in the world and time. Things will break, not just bones.

*Jump Piece* was the last work Hsieh did in his natal country, Taiwan, and the first performance or action piece of his career. Before it, he painted. After it, he flew, fleeing Taiwan to America, sailed really, "jumping ship," as he put it, and defecting, while he was doing mandatory service in the Taiwanese equivalent of the merchant marines. To say he "flew" is not right, then, for his life's flight was really about jumping and jumping really about landing, jumping ship so as to land in a new world. This is unlike Klein, who appears to believe that humans are not earthbound but can indeed fly, aerial men who need not worry about their landing. When Hsieh jumped, he didn't know where he would land. For many years, he lived in America as an unrecognized illegal. It was indeed the new world into which he landed, and about the only thing that can be said with certainty about beginning life as a defector without documents in a new world is that it will be new, ever and again new, each moment.

As a precursor to a flight that is in truth a jumping ship, *Jump Piece* is very much about landing, and landing is no light matter. I'd like to leap into my days (Klein), not just fall into them, but Hsieh's earthbound jumps remind me of the facts: every heartfelt leap also falls to earth. That gives me pause.

Hsieh's jump points out that how you land makes a big difference in how you take the fall: you don't want to crash but to land in such a way that you can walk on. Perhaps the word for that is gracefully, not catastrophically (Hsieh) and not insouciantly (Klein) but gracefully: like a dancer. Kierkegaard saw that. As much as he was fascinated by leaping, what commands my attention now is his consideration of the landing more than of the leap, considerations that he organizes explicitly around the figure of the dancer and his graceful movements. Kierkegaard saw that the passionate leap is in fact a way of coming down to earth and landing. Eternal highs are not what the leap of faith is about, then, and anyone who tells you that passion is endlessly euphoric is selling you a cheap and easy version. All who leap also land. The leap of faith, I see more clearly now, is meant to be that: a way to come down to earth, gracefully.

Reflecting on leaping under the pseudonym Johannes di Silentio in one of his most famous writings, *Fear and Trembling*, Kierkegaard identifies two types of dancers—he also calls them knights. The first dancer, the knight of infinity, leaps perfectly, a consummate dancer of ballet. The second, the knight of faith, leaps only to land, walking on in the most pedestrian of ordinary realities.

It is supposed to be the most difficult feat for a ballet dancer to leap into a specific posture in such a way that he never once strains for the posture but in the very leap assumes the posture. Perhaps there is no ballet dancer who can do it—but this knight does it. . . . The knights of infinity are ballet dancers and have elevation. They make the upward movement and come down again, and this, too, is not an unhappy diversion and is not unlovely to see. But every time they come down they are not able to assume the posture immediately, they waver for a moment. . . . To be able to come down in such a way that instantaneously one seems to stand and to walk, to change the leap into life into walking, absolutely to express the sublime in the pedestrian—only that knight [of faith] can do it, and this is the one and only marvel. (41)

Two types of dancers then: the ballet dancer and the pedestrian.

Inhabitant of the infinite, the perfect ballet dancer hovers just off the floor, on toes that touch the floor only tangentially. He is scarcely ever landing, seeming always instead to be leaping and leaping effortlessly, immediately into a pose, as if never in motion or moving toward that pose. This is what makes the ballet dancer transcendent, an inhabitant of the infinite: ethereal, he hovers in a pose set above finite reality and succeeds in leaving the earth behind.

The perfect ballet dancer marries leaping and composure, each erasing the other. If I were to imagine the movement of one, it would be like watching images taken out of a filmstrip, abstracted from the stretch of time that distends them. Each frame would be a perfect pose, none transitional or transitory, none on the way or reaching for a pose, none seeking or searching, each a moment without momentum. A series of perfectly composed poses, the leaping is erased, and with it perhaps the passion, too—a dancer whose heart is not in it?

The second dancer, the knight of faith, higher for Kierkegaard than the knight of infinity, is the one who lands. His leap
belongs to the pedestrian, Kierkegaard says, the ordinary walk
through everyday life, not to the *prima donna* of ballet. It becomes
a way of landing and walking on in the finite world, alongside
everybody else also walking along. The knight of faith goes about
his business, conducts his affairs, and tackles the projects of
everyday life. He might have a family, a husband or wife. He
loves others and has friends and associates, partners, business and
otherwise. He has a job, perhaps as a professor or maybe a tax
collector, Kierkegaard suggests, and things to do, obligations to
fulfill in order to be responsible to these positions in life. He
keeps lists like the rest of us of what needs doing, long lists that
only grow longer as items get lined out over the course of the day.
He knows, I suspect, that each time a call is made he will receive
two more to answer in response, that the to-do list grows precisely by the doing of what makes it shrink, that what gets lined
out shows up again at the bottom of the list in need of doing
again . . . and again. It's tiring, the tedium often overcomes me.
But when five o'clock comes around and the work is over, he has
not lost heart: he thinks of the "special hot meal [waiting] for
him when he comes home—for example, roast lamb's head with
vegetables," even though he and his family lack the means for so
delectable a feast and his wife does not cook much. "If he meets
a kindred soul" on this walk home, Kierkegaard continues, "he
would go on talking all the way to Østerport about this delicacy
with a passion befitting a restaurant operator." It is a mundane,
pedestrian world through which the knight of faith walks, talking with others like a restauranteur passionate about everyday
concerns such as shopping, cooking, feeding others, and so on.
This makes it "impossible to distinguish him from the rest of the
crowd. . . . In the evening, he smokes his pipe; seeing him one

would swear it was the butcher" (39–40). Knights of faith are therefore "likely to disappoint, for externally they have a strik-ing resemblance to bourgeois philistinism. . . . To see the [knight of faith] makes one think of a pen-pusher" (38–39). He is no mas-ter of ballet and hardly a *prima donna*, just an ordinary walker like all the other passersby in the crowd immersed in everyday concerns that occupy all of us alike, and yet he does not seem dis-heartened by it, any of it.

Why? How? He goes through it in good cheer, every day. How does he do it? How does he find the heart for it? I, like Johannes de Silentio, the pseudonym who signs the book, can't imagine where it comes from. When I try, my thoughts are drawn back to the leap. Remember the leap. His pedestrian walk, Kierkegaard tells me, is the landing of a leap, a passionate move-ment, in other words. The passion is not erased from the days of his everyday if I remember the leap. He finds himself there, "by virtue of the absurd."

It turns out that the leap is not into the void from mundane life, it's a leap into everyday life *from the void*. To have landed in everyday life by dropping into it from the groundless void—that is a terrifying thought to those who think that everything needs a cause or reason justifying why it is and is as it is; everyday life seems to dissolve in terrifying unreality and nonnecessity when it loses ground and purpose. But it doesn't have to be only ter-rifying or cause for despair.

The knight of faith has no grounds for existing on the ground he does. If this is not despair, it is passion. He comes into his pedestrian existence passionately, by a leap, dropping into it by dropping out, out of the blue, as it were. The knight of faith has found the heart for this abysmal ground of ordinary life not to be cause for despair. He is not disappointed to have landed on ordinary ground after leaping groundlessly but "changes the leap into life into walking, absolutely expresses the sublime in the pedestrian" (41). Having dropped into the world groundlessly, being there is something to wonder at and about. The ordinary has become eventful when it is reached by landing in it from the void, without grounds. Abysmal, yes, but the absurdity of the ground on which he walks makes the ordinary a wonder to the knight of faith, not a problem but something to wonder about.

That's the benefit of remembering the void out of which we leap into our ordinary days. Such thoughts might make it harder to carry on gracefully; they might make one stumble and despair; but the knight of faith has the heart for the grace.

Do I? That is the question asked by the uncomprehending signatory of *Fear and Trembling*, Johannes di Silentio, he who is so admiring of yet appalled by that knight's graceful walk: Where do I find the heart for that pedestrian existence, he seems to be asking throughout this book.

Though perhaps obvious, the importance of how you land struck me while watching a dance performance one night in April 2019, a little over six months after I had come home from the hospital. In fact, it was my eleven-year-old son's dance performance—assuring me it doesn't take an expert to land gracefully, and the prima donna of classical ballet is not even the best model. The kids could do it, I saw, the kids doing contemporary dance. One of the signature movements of the studio where he dances is the roll. Young people learn they can land safely by rolling. Fluid rolling, roll into a standing pose—or rather roll into walking, since you don't hold the pose. The roll is in this way, I saw, also a way to leap into the fall and its landing. For these young people, graceful and rolling are mutual qualifiers, which is not how I, uneducated to be sure, imagine the ballet dancer, who does not roll but is always leaping while ever composed, ever in the air, light and levitating, and only on the ground tangentially, on the tips of his toes. Not so the youth. They rolled, which means they spent a lot of time on the floor, not just lifting off but grounded, a status that would be failure if we were meant for flight, like birds, angels, Yves Klein, or an airplane, it was for them a condition to explore. Learning to roll on the floor, they learned to move gracefully on the ground.

Klein leaped but did not fall.

Hsieh leaped and fell but did not roll.

There are important lessons to be learned from rolling. My son's instructor, who also teaches at a nearby college, tried to teach me some. She tells me that it, like dance, is about your relation to the floor, the ground toward which you fall when you are dragged down, as you inevitably are, by the everyday, common fact of gravity. Work with the floor, then, she tells me; roll with it, as they say. It puts a bottom to your falling, and if you don't learn to get to the bottom, to let yourself hit bottom, and be with it, your fall will be endless.

People who roll can fall more exquisitely, and they can rise to walk on the ground. This might be why it is the way to land gracefully. Rolling with it, then, is perhaps a measure of grace when falling defines us. While "roll with it" sounds like insouciance or carefree acquiescence, for these dancers, it is not. The insouciant doesn't care: reality being immaterial, the material being unreal, he doesn't feel the weight, the tug of gravity; the floor is of no concern to him, therefore he is above all that, levitating. It's different with the dancer whose movement is defined by falling: he feels the tug of gravity and, drawn toward something and somewhere else, has nagging questions about the grave matter of his landing—as I have to imagine Hsieh did, too, when he jumped. This dancer cares about the floor, takes it into consideration, and works with it to roll so as to stand and walk on, dancing. Nobody who sees such a dance falling and rising, careful about its relation to the floor, would describe it as insouciant.

This movement, my son's instructor continued, belongs to a form of dance that has departed from classical ballet's insistence on a certain kind of center and centering. The ballet teacher tells you to remain centered in yourself, to find and adhere to a center in you. There is no falling, or at least there shouldn't be. Posing is the aim, and the pose holds when it is centered. Disturbance, on this model, comes from outside, external forces that push the pose off center again. The centered dancer of ballet triumphs over these externalities, neutralizes them so as to remain immune from the mutability they impose on the ballet dancer and his body. His movement, then, is his own. It is initiated by forces inside the dancer, the autonomous dancer, a self-possessed prima donna, a master. Contemporary dancers, by contrast, fall, she says. At the studio where my son dances, their movement often looks to me like they are falling into it. They fall always because, depending on what teacher you follow, there is no center, the center is not in them, or there are multiple centers tugging in a field of forces. Perhaps the simplest way I found to think about it was to see that the dancer falls because the center in them is not the only center. There is a center out there, down there even, bigger than I, in the ground beneath the floor. The earth pulls us down. The dancer senses it.

That sensation is the feel of gravity.

Sensing the gravity of things gives birth to the weight of my being.

Being me is weighty.

Weight falls.

I fall.

.

.

.

Under the sway of their gravity, we are attracted to things and move in their direction; they are attractive, we say. The tug of their gravity gives life to something in us—we call it "weight." Our lives take on weight by force of that gravity as we fall toward things. The weight is mine, then, and there is a center of it in me, but the weight of my being and my center are born as a response to the other center whose weight I feel first as the draw of gravity, the attraction of things. One of the more unsettling implications of all this is, of course, that feeling the attraction of things and the world means taking on weight: it's a burden to be drawn to the everyday world of things, perhaps even more so the more attractive they are.

This is what it is like to take things to heart. When you care about matters and respond to their gravity, they give weight to life, a weight that tugs on you and even drags you down. The heart, organ for the sensation of the gravity of ordinary things, is where the attraction is felt but also the drag. The logic of the heart is the logic of gravity, I concluded while watching the children dance. It's a grave logic, Karl Ove Knausgaard is right: "The heart beats and then it does not. That's it." But though grave, the logic of gravity is not without grace. I saw the children give it a try in April as they leaped and landed in movements of graceful rolling. When skilled dancers take on gravity and the weight that is born in them of it, burdensome facts become graceful appearances. Their leap into falling is joyous. Klein got that right. We do want to leap like Klein, we want levity in our life, but if the levity is not to be empty, it has to have some weight— which means it will not ascend endlessly, will fall and rise again, beating on, until eventually it falls finally and will not ascend ever again. When the exhilaration of the leap is hearty and not just titillating or gleeful, it feels the tug and pull of gravity drawing it back as it rises.

Bas Jan Ader (1942–disappeared 1975?) also practiced an art of gravity and made work of falling, a series known simply as the *Fall* pieces (1970–71).[7] He is noted in passing in the same book by Adrian Heathfield where Hsieh's *Jump Piece* is discussed. Reading more about his career, I began to take heart from what I saw in his works. They are brilliant manifestations of heart, showing it or making it appear in the midst of falling. As I struggled to recover mine, his was all the more apparent to me. Sensing the appearance of his, I began to feel my own. The heart he made manifest in his work was the one that came to life in me, the one I call mine the one he manifested.

Known like Klein and Hsieh for his life works, Ader's *Fall* pieces are his most iconic. One of the more famous is a slow-motion film of him falling off the roof of his house, *Fall 1, Los Angeles* (1970). Beginning with him seated at rest in a chair at the peak of the roof, the work involves him tilting slightly off-center and tipping over. He tumbles, as you would expect for earth-bound mortals pulled in response to gravity, down the high-sloping roof until his fall arrives at the less steeply sloped roof of an attached porch below. Our hearts go out to him, and there is a brief moment where we hope, imagining he might catch himself and stop the fall, but what we hope might be an end is just a pause: he catches himself only momentarily and continues to tumble, then drops over the edge, landing in a thicket of bushes that surround the house. A critic for the *Los Angeles Times* described his roll as tumbling "with the awkward grace that recalls Buster Keaton's antics."

I laughed out loud when I saw the awkwardly graceful roll but caught myself. Ader's fall is funny up until the point you realize he will land. It would, I think, take a certain heartlessness to keep laughing. Unlimited laughter seems more appropriate for ecstatic leaps like Yves Klein's, when the laughter can be endless because the leap is into a void where all matters are immaterial and nothing ever falls. For earthbound beings with a heart, however, endless laughter is not a possibility. To be sure, there is something comical about Ader's *Fall* pieces, but these works of falling, like those of Keaton, have a gravity to them. It makes us catch our breath and smile ruefully before we laugh ourselves all the way to death—saving us from endless laughter, which I don't find funny after a while anyway, I don't want to have made my lifetime a joke. It is apt, then, that a (presumably) posthumous exhibition of Ader's work was titled *Bas Jan Ader: Suspended Between Laughter and Tears* (Nichols Gallery and Lenzner Family Gallery, Pitzer College, 2010).

Is that where the heart is found? Does following your heart mean finding yourself somewhere between laughter and tears? The slim smile that pushes its way up in me comes from there, somewhere between grief and glee, between succumbing to the tragedy of our falling lives and affirming, with insouciance, the bliss of an immaterial life.

A truly hearty laugh, then, is in fact one that falls silent and turns into a thin smile before it comes to its end. One might say, in French, Simon Critchley points out, that my *rire* (laughing) turns into a *sourire* (smiling, literally *sou-rire*, sub-laughter),[8] a diminutive, minor laugh in a minor key, a smile that laughs quietly, silently even, not loudly because not at all sure it is laughing at funny things. In a world measured by the logic of the heart, the unrestrained laugh, only light with buoyancy, pure glee, is too much;

a grimace, only heavy with effort, too little; a reticent smile more to the point. It is what Critchley, citing Samuel Beckett's *Watt* in the epigraph to his book *On Humour*, calls *mirthless laughter*, the "laugh that laughs—silence please—at that which is unhappy."

The reserved smile of a mirthless laugh shows that I am taking grave matters seriously but without being crushed by the weight born in me when I sense their gravity. It is sad, after all, Ader's fall. It's not just funny, but sad. The reality of that sadness stirs my heart, resonates in it as an unhappiness of my own, and yet, despite it all—despite the gravity of the inevitable end, the grave anticipated in every moment of the work; and despite the sadness inside me, the sad weight of the world taken in me— despite it all, a smile rises up. That smile, not at all straightforward and somewhat crooked, is a mixed-up, confused expression, hard to bear and hard to interpret. It shows a feeling that might not fit neatly into the popular categories of either positive or negative emotion—what does positive psychology make of this, I wonder?—but it is the expression of a being with a heart, one who can be out of tune with the world that nevertheless resonates in it, smiling at what is sad, indeed at the sadness it, too, feels.

Critchley says that such a smile is consoling: "this smile . . . does not bring unhappiness, but rather elevation and liberation, the lucidity of consolation. This is why melancholy animals that we are, human beings are also the most cheerful" (111). If one thinks according to the logic of the heart the smile that Critchley rightly says is consolation is born in con-dolation, condolence, that is. Ader tumbling down the roof is a grave matter. It will hurt when he lands, and I, my heart going out to him, even though I know better, certain that it is just a stunt, feel his pain and am pained myself, too. The smile that slowly, tentatively crosses my face does not show cruelty or indifference toward him nor evidence an unlimited joy and confidence for me. Is it the expression of the heart that leaps up in me in response to the descent of Ader's? I believe so—an expression of condolence, then? One that also consoles?

Confronting this expression of my heart must be, for friends and family, colleagues and others, as hard to bear as it is to interpret. It must be a bit like my own encounter with the cryptic smile of the Hindu gods seen in the sculpture I share with students in my "Introduction to Religion" class. There are pictures in the back of the book we use, an old one, out of date by standards more contemporary than mine, Heinrich Zimmer's *Myth and Symbol in Indian Art and Civilization*. I am looking at one of the god Shiva now.

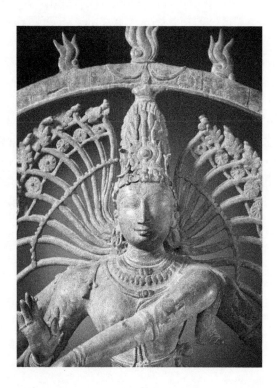

These divine smiles, Zimmer says, are to be seen as coming from a vision of all-consuming voids and void-consuming alls that arise and pass away in cycles older than the universe itself, cycles to which the gods too must submit. We are supposed to see the gods, he continues, pointing to the truth that individual life in these whirling cycles is like an ant in a parade of ants marching on stage against the backdrop of cosmic eons, as small and insignificant as that. The gods do not take on the weight of that fact with a grimace, however. They see the truth of tumbling through lives in a vast, barren and indifferent cosmos in which individual action makes no ultimate difference, but they do not see that truth only to grin and bear it, smiling through clenched teeth as it were. That is not the divine way to be. The gods' smile is instead serene, composed, a being at peace that comes from being attuned to this play of the cosmos. It is a playful smile, Zimmer assures me.

Students don't often agree with Zimmer. There is a hint of irony in the smile, the students say, not exactly a smirk but the gods seem to know something they are not telling us, some secret that lets them be at peace and live divinely. I don't disagree with the students. I often feel a bit as if god and the gods are laughing at me and my heartfelt worries, even the ones about my heart. Theirs is anything but the smile of condolence, it seems, and my thoughts anything but consoling. Insecure, I cannot help but suspect the gods are insincere and mocking, not just playful but playing with me, like cats. My smile at Ader's tumble and fall might look that way to others, those who do not have their ear to my heart. It is not supposed to. I really don't know something special that I am keeping secret; the experience of heart surgery did not confide in me some secret I am not sharing. I, too, am trying to figure out where that smile with life's falling comes from. I have come now to think that it comes from a place suspended between laughter and tears where the heart and its grave logic are found to play.

Another piece in which I found a brilliant manifestation of heart is Ader's *Broken Fall (Organic)* (1971). Here the art of gravity is given even greater sway. Eliminating the moment of rest that opens *Fall 1* (where he is seated on a chair), the work starts with Ader out on a limb, dangling from a tree that stretches over a small creek or canal. Swinging restlessly from the beginning, he hangs on as long as he can, but he cannot forever and so he falls, landing in the dark waters below. In contrast to *Fall 1*, the fall that consummates this work is not initiated by the artist and his power (it is not the leap of a master of ballet) but by the exhaustion of his power to maintain any center, even a moving one. It ends with him slumped on the banks of the creek, still not out of the water, still not fully ashore, but it's over. The film lasts only a short 01:44, but it is an agonizingly long short 01:44. You know the end will come, but you don't know when. I sat on the edge of my seat, with him on the verge of his collapse, holding my breath as he tries to hang on.

There is a beauty to the way he sways as he hangs on, adjusting his weight again and again in response to the pull of gravity. It is not the beauty of a perfect pose. His composure lost before he ever finds it, Ader has not found his center. It's more like he is ever seeking it or ever finding it and losing it, trying to right himself over and over. To be sure, it is a jerky, hesitant movement that kicks and sways, but I find it beautiful and am attracted to it.

I can see that his heart is in it, but there is a gap, an inequality, between his heart and his strength—the former exceeding the latter, his heart greater than his power to achieve, succeed, or be wholly effective. That's why he moves in these fits and starts, hesitancies and spasms. Out on a limb, he wants to hang on, he tries to, his heart is in it, but he can do so only so long. This makes for the tension that is ever seeking to right itself by swinging, and for the beauty, too, that I see in that swinging. That's life. It's beautiful. It's not steady, though, it swings, constantly steadying itself because always unsteady. There is a balance: it just swings as one hangs out on a limb.

Out on a limb, you can live that swinging balance beautifully. Ader does.

But you cannot hold on always or forever. It will crash, break, from time to time, and finally one day, finally, the swinging will stop, and you will fall straight down.

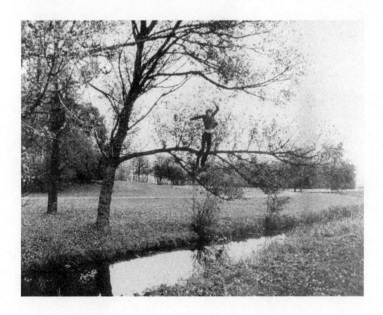

Ader falls. It's not even the case that he released his grip. It would be nice to say he let go, but he just can't hold on any longer. Gravity wins. It always does.

But the heart remains. Ader lays it bare. I glimpsed it already as he swings from the limb while the strength to hang on slowly fades, but I see it naked, as it were, near the end when his strength is exhausted and he falls, without wanting to, while still wanting to hang on. His heart has taken him there, to a point where the heart remains beyond the strength it takes to do what he has the heart to do. All that remains is the heart, a very fragile, exposed heart, absent the power to hang on. And it falls. This is what makes Ader's work so poignant for me: it exposes the heart it takes to hang on by removing the power to do so.

I didn't see this until it was over. It was only after I saw it laid bare in its fall, slumped on the side of the canal and expiring with the heavy sigh of the end, that I felt the heart made manifest. Too late, and unlike in films which can be run again, am I learning the lessons of the heart's logic. There are no do-overs in life, no chances to rewind and repeat what is past, see it again, do it again. These moments when I sit at the window or my desk, looking on, imagining possible lives and meaningful projects without having the heart to throw myself into them . . . they are gone. I saw too late the heart it takes for that leap, found the heart for it after the time and the times were gone. "Late for the love of my life," they say in that song by the Lumineers that I often hear playing in Claire's room and Oscar's room.

# 8

## HEARTFELT

*One day I will go to Teshima Island in the Japanese archipelago and visit* Les archives du coeur. *The archives were installed there in 2010 by the artist Christian Boltanski. A shrine as much as an archive,* Les archives du coeur *holds Boltanski's collection of heartbeats. A good place to find one, therefore, and I have been looking for a while now. Using up to date technologies, you can browse the archive and listen to the heart of tens of thousands of individuals who have used similar technologies to record theirs and leave it in Boltanski's collection. A good place to put yours, too, then, for you can also record the beat of the one you call mine and leave your heart, or at least a piece of it, in Boltanski's ever-growing collection.*

*The initial deposits to Boltanski's collection were made at locations throughout the world, then relocated to Teshima. The first came from a man in Sweden, who also asked to include the heartbeat of his dog. Six thousand other Swedish heartbeats were included in this first installment. Boltanski went on from there to collect a global diversity that includes heartbeats from Chile, Botswana, Korea, every nation in Europe, and more. Many were collected at sites where his art was installed, one of the most notable being* Personnes, *presented at the Grand Palais in Paris in early 2010, the same year as* Les archives du coeur *opened.* Personnes *arranged the abandoned clothing of anon-*

*ymous individuals in piles on the floor of the Grand Palais but without the heart that made those individual lives live, an absence made present by the ambient sound of a heartbeat pulsing in the vast hall.*

*People seem eager to add their own to Boltanski's collection. A report on* Personnes *notes that one Sunday in January 2010, the line for leaving one's heart in the archive was an hour long.[1] Boltanski is clearly onto something in his solicitation of our hearts: lots of us appear to be looking to find and give ours. There were more than twenty thousand heartbeats in the initial deposit to the archives on Teshima, and it continues to grow.*

*When I go there, I will record the beat of the heart I call mine, leaving it alongside all the others in the archives. It will be my new heart, the changed one, the repaired one, or perhaps by that time, my new new heart, one with a new new valve and updated expiration date, but in any case, one without the pistol shot backfire that accompanied the heart I was born with. I almost wrote "the one that accompanied my heart from the beginning." But which beginning and when did it all begin? These are the questions my heart poses these days. Did it begin a couple Septembers ago in 2018? Is this one mine, or is the first one mine? Will there be another next one? Did I miss the chance to archive my own by coming after the fact of its supplement . . . and before the fact of its supplement? Which one will be the last? Do I really want to know?*

It's just a dream. Going to Teshima Island to find the heart to get on with mine is just an idea that came to me while I was reading a book, *La vie possible de Christian Boltanski,* as part of research for a course I teach on religion and secularity. I haven't ever been there.

I did, however, visit *Pulse* by Rafael Lozano-Hemmer at the Hirshhorn Museum in Washington, DC, an easy drive of three hours. Browsing the news one day, the work attracted my attention for the obvious reason: its title referred to a heartbeat at a time when I was listening very carefully for one of my own. It was November, and I was just coming back to everyday life. Reading more about *Pulse*, I learned that it was an interactive installation in which visitors' heartbeats were used to create audible and visible effects in the surrounding environment of the gallery: projected images, lights that flickered, wave patterns in shallow pools, and so on.

Work was being made with a heart, and work with a heart is being made, this is what I am looking for, I thought to myself. Proof that you have a heart, displayed right there on the wall or in the pool at your feet. Evidence that the heart has an effect on the world, right there where all can see. Doubting my own, I was drawn in.

By an odd coincidence, the show happened to be installed in Washington at the same time as I had planned to take my eleven-year-old son to the city to see the New York Giants play the Washington Redskins. He claims to be a Giants fan. Our plans had been made in August for his birthday before any and all planning was interrupted by the decision for heart surgery. The plans remained in suspense following surgery when my to-do lists were cleared. Actually going on the trip depended on my finding the heart for it, and I couldn't. The same could be said of a projected visit to *Pulse*. I imagined visiting but couldn't find the heart for it. Something happened, however, that changed things. I don't know if it was *Pulse* that put the game back on a list labeled "to-do" or the game that put *Pulse* on such a list, but it happened, I did it, I threw myself into it, and we made a day of it, two in fact.

*Pulse* gathered three pieces from a series Lozano-Hemmer had made over several years. Using devices that capture finger-print and heart rate, the first piece, *Pulse Index*, projects images of both onto an opposite wall where they appear together in a single frame on a grid. The heartbeat and finger of the last five hundred or so participants remain on the wall until another adds her data to the screen. I could not escape the sense that we had become taggers, leaving our heart as signatures like so much graffiti on the wall for all to see—or not just a signature, more like a stamp, an image impressed on the screen by the activity of my living body. We all want to make an impression, it seemed to say, and here is a chance to do it and moreover do it in front of others. Oscar, my son, enjoyed himself while he participated. It's evident in the photographs.

In the second piece, *Pulse Tank*, a visitor would insert her finger in a plastic tube where a sensor detects her pulse. The beat of her heart, magnified technologically to the point that she can

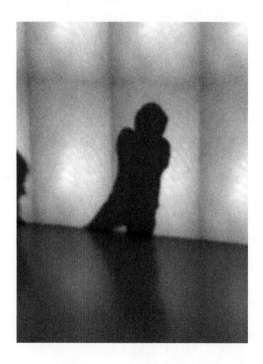

hear it, drums loud and strong, and with its beating, blows air through the tube into a pool of water where it makes waves with each beat. Light projected over the surface of the water shows these waves as reflections on the opposite wall of the room. Seeing your pulse materialize in waves and patterns is an arresting sight. It was hard not to stand captivated by the image. Evidence that it is not a lost cause after all. I enjoyed watching myself and others, and I have memorable photographs of my son.

The third and final piece is *Pulse Room*. Hundreds of light bulbs hang in rows from the ceiling of a comfortably curving, long gallery. Visitors queue up at the far end, waiting to place their finger on a panel that detects their heartbeat. When it is your turn and your finger is on the button, the beat of your heart is amplified so that all of us throughout the room can hear. That

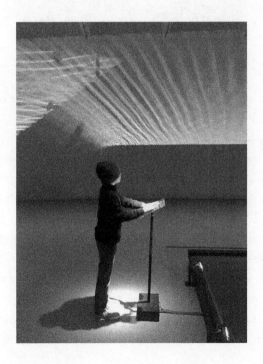

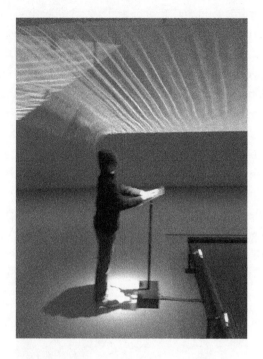

beat is also located visually in the first lightbulb of each row. With each subsequent beat of your heart, the first bulb passes the previous beat to the next bulb in line, which now beats with it and passes on the beat it contained to the third bulb, and so on and so on, filling the room with ever more light and sound. There is little to no harmony as the beating and flickering is translated from one bulb to the next, only an increasing roar and dazzle, until the room is filled with one steady glare and one steady blare, then it's over, and the next visitor has a turn.

The installation was popular and successful. Apparently I am not the only one looking for a heart. It was as if much of America was searching for signs that they still had one. *Pulse* did not frustrate those seekers. Evidence of heartbeats materialized everywhere. Proof that you have a heart was found in all three rooms. "Look," the seekers can say, "mine can ripple the surface and stir up a still pool. My heartbeat has an effect: it can power a cascade of light and sound that will make you blink and hold your ears." People want to make waves; all the better if they can do it with their hearts. People want reassurance that their heart matters: they could see that it does in the waves it makes. That's important. In this day and age when it's hard to have a heart, it can help to have a time and space where it is made visible and moreover visible before everybody that we do indeed have one. Public recognition of something in common always makes it easier to admit you in particular have it too. *Pulse* is doing a good thing, then, letting us all feel confident admitting we have a heart.

But I was disappointed. It was as if the heart had been put to work in the production of entertaining images, "cool" effects, and dazzling evidence, while work with a heart was not being made. Thunderous appearances of quiet beats, does that really show how it feels to have one? Does the ability to make waves really prove that we have a heart? Waves are on the surface, after all, hearts much deeper. Lozano-Hemmer's success in making the heart visible and audible hid the heart that made the work. The lights and the roar magnify what is faint in us, and I applaud this work of magnification: to magnify is to praise, after all, and I am persuaded that the work of the heart is in need of praise. But this sort of magnification, making it so big you can't miss it, making it so bright you see it without looking—this sort of magnification is not a magnification of that small thing, that thing which can by definition be missed and is to be, one day, definitively missed because definitively missing. This is more like fattening it up, making it all the more ready for easy access and consumption, and then it is no longer the small thing in need of magnification that is being magnified.

The truth is, I find now that I have lost it, having a heart is not a matter of having an effect, not a matter of making waves. *Pulse* risks making the heart too much a part of the noisy public place we call "the world that counts." In that world, it itself becomes loud and noisy in order to prove that it, too, counts like all the rest—evident, to be sure, and evident to all, but the drive for public evidence that my heart matters risks making matters of the heart disappear or else making them appear blown all out of proportion in entertaining drama like I see in the tabloids and talk shows. We need other times and spaces to find the heart I am looking for.

I left *Pulse* disappointed with what I had found and frustrated in my searching. The heart I was looking for was not here, and here was not where I wanted to put my heart. I went back to dreaming about Teshima Island.

Teshima Island is a quiet place far away. Quiet places, places at a remove, let things like the heart come forward as it is: faint. Nobody wants to admit publicly to being faint or fainting, but hearts are and do, they grow faint and fainter and then faint, the one I call mine will eventually and forever. In my dream of Teshima Island, having a heart will be a much quieter affair than at *Pulse*, and yet it will be magnified.

Boltanski speaks directly to this magnification when he identifies what he says is one of the most important things art can do: "A small thing can become very, very grand. A little painting on a wall can take up the entire wall just like a big one."[2] This is what it means *to magnify*. Much of Boltanski's art is characterized by it. He collects "tiny things" in vitrines, hangs them on walls, or puts them on pedestals—things such as sugar cubes, passport photos, locks of hair, toy soldiers, votive candles, and eyeglasses, for instance. Hearts, too. The things in these collections are not made big or loud but afforded a time and space where, though small and faint, they can loom large, be seen up close and, raised up on the pedestal of art, be glorified, praised. *The Dead Swiss* is a good example. Rephotographed images taken at random from the obituaries of an off-market, provincial Swiss newspaper are framed, placed on shelves, and leaned against the wall of the gallery, where a clip lamp on each is the only illumination in the room. These nondescript lives lived far from the center of things, these lives lacking in world-historical significance, small in the grand scheme of things—these "tiny things" are magnified when raised up by Boltanski's monumental work. So, too, I imagine, at Teshima Island. There, I will find not only an archive of hearts but also an altar or shrine dedicated to their magnification.

*Les archives du coeur* comprises three rooms. The first is a listening room, in which you become attuned to your heart by listening to one. The room itself is long and dark, with a single bulb on the ceiling at one end. The bulb blinks steadily to the tune of a magnified heartbeat from Boltanski's collection. The rhythmic beat affords only intermittent glimpses of the room and others in it. I am in the dark. Blind and groping. Mirrors mounted along the walls diffuse the light of the beating heart along the length of the hall. Visitors describe their own heart, itself like a mirror, beating with the rhythm now running through them. I am finally attuned, a heart found leaps up inside me drawn out by the beat I have been following.

The second room is a recording room where white-coated attendants assist visitors in archiving their heart. The attendants are frequently likened to medical personnel, but I imagine them equally as deacons or acolytes whose office is to minister to the pilgrims who have come so far at such great expense to offer their heart. Because it's hard to have a heart, hard to find one, and hard to know where to put it, we need such ministers. They are rare today.

In addition to helping with the technology, the assistants also take your money, collect the fee you pay for giving your heart to Boltanski's archive. Swindlers? Is this really just a confidence game played by a swindler who is tricking you out of your money by promising to archive your heartbeat forever? Shouldn't we steer clear of seducers like this, who play on our hearts and our hearts' desires? Those who spend too much time listening to their heart are likely to fall for it.

At least one critic declares such suspicions. "The whole project is supposedly humanitarian (an archive of human heartbeats) so, while I was in the building, why did I have a constant feeling that the artist was trying to rip us off in as many ways as he could?" she writes, and then continues. "First of all, admission was ¥500 instead of the usual ¥300 for paying artworks (even though, personally, I didn't have to pay—I really did love that Press Pass). And it got worse, because if you wanted your heartbeat to be recorded you had to pay ¥1500!"[3] This critic clearly suspects deceptions and seducers and steels her heart against them. She wants to be certain that it is a good deal before leaping in, and she would rather negotiate the terms of a settlement agreeable to both parties before she will even consider offering her heart. "Mr. Boltanski, if you want my heartbeat in your archives," she writes, "it's you who should pay me and not the other way around. Sure, I don't have to be greedy, tell me about the human dimension, the legacy for future generations and all those things, and maybe, just maybe, if you use the right words, I may accept to let you record it for free. But making me pay to help you get richer and more famous and getting nothing in return?" On guard against giving without getting something equal, this critic keeps her heart to herself. No deal. She won't fall for it.

But you don't go to the island of your dreams with your critical faculties intact. Boltanski has made it a work of the heart, and that proves foolish business, the critic is right, but its foolishness might not be a reason not to do the work. You cannot do the work of the heart unless you stop trying to sort out the problem of who is giving and who is taking in the relation that it is. Paying the fee to make an offering of your heart, it's not clear who is the maker of the work, who is really serving whom, who is giving and who is taking—not unlike the psychoanalytic relation. Someone might be taking advantage of you, but a heart is open and not made of stone, its work therefore exposed to exploitation, danger, and betrayal. Such betrayal, painful no doubt, betrays the openness of having a heart. Only in the logic of the heart does our weakness for such exploitation not count against it, even if we must acknowledge it with sadness. This logic is not adhered to by the suspicious critic, and not following it, she will not find her heart in Boltanski's archive. She will go home without one— because she wouldn't put hers in it, much less leave it there.

The third room is the archive itself. It is a listening room that overlooks the inland sea one has crossed to reach the island. You sit comfortably at a computer terminal with headphones on and search Boltanski's collection, scanning the names in a long list looking for the heart you seek and listening to it quietly. Maybe that of someone you know, a lost friend, your grandmother. Maybe someone you wish you knew, a celebrity, a historically important figure, a desired friend. Maybe just a name chosen at random from the mass of individuals with beating hearts like yours.

There is something impersonal about this intimacy, and something intimate about this impersonal encounter. All the others, dead or alive, reduced to just the beat of their heart, what could be more intimate to them, more intimately their own than their heart, yet it says nothing about what they did or do with their life, the color of their skin or distinguishing anatomical features, who they loved and who they made love to, their accomplishments and their failures. It's the inside-out of Boltanski's earlier work, *Inventaires*, for example, where the personal effects of individuals—toothbrush, eyeglasses, favorite books, and so on—are arranged in vitrines or boxes, the things that constitute a life gathered together absent the heart a person put into living the life with those things. The person has been taken out of the personal effects. The effects remain, the effects that individualize us and identify us as who we are, but they remain in the absence of the "cause," the "person," whatever it is, that make those effects personal, effects of a living individual. In *Les archives du coeur* it is the inverse: you hear nothing that would identify the individual whose most intimate intimacy you nevertheless listen to in your ignorance of who it is; you hear nothing about her world, her history, or the personal effects and things that surrounded her and made up her life. All you hear is the heart she called mine.

What is it you are listening to when the things and personal effects, the experiences and accomplishments, remain unknown? What is it you attend to when you don't know the identity of who it is you are listening to? The heart you hear is the register of her care and concern for those things, its beat the intimate inward response to the coming and going, the arising and passing away, of all the things, people and projects, that concerned her—her loves, her love. Attending to it, you don't know who you are listening to, yet you are as close as possible to what is closest to them.

What is it in you that listens? What is it in you that attends? My heart?

A true heart-to heart, then, on Teshima Island? Mine leaps to life with the one it hears. Having one that is mine is the only way to find theirs.

It's just a dream. It might be true. Don't be so suspicious. This is one archive that rewards the naive and maybe even ignorant searcher.

I realize that in this dream of Teshima Island, I vacillate, saying sometimes that I am looking to find my heart and at other times that I am listening to my heart. It's worth calling attention to that oscillation. It is as if I am looking to find a heart by listening to it, following its beat so as to find it out there in the distance somewhere on an island in the dark or befogged seas. What have I lost, then, if I am already listening to my heart, and what does it mean to find it if I am listening to one I call mine? If I listen to my heart, I might find it, out there, wherever it is, because mine is not in me, what is most intimately mine, my heart, is outside me, ever to be found and therefore in a sense constitutively lost. In a certain strange way, then, finding the one I call mine means being found by another that I listen to. It finds the heart in me? One I can call mine is found by it? Listening to it is a way to find it? A logic that holds because it is lost? Lost, it can only be found by following it while listening. I follow what is lost, following my heart means following the lost thing I listen to? The heart's logic is perplexing.

All this is not unrelated to the fact that I also oscillate between saying the archive is where I will find a heart and where I will leave mine. Is Teshima where I am looking to take heart or where I am looking to put one? More and more, it seems as if this ambiguity also comes from a paradox true to life: I will find heart by putting mine in it, and putting my heart in it is the only way to take heart. And yet if it takes heart, soon enough it will all be taken, and I will have none.

Following *my* heart, too. There is a paradox in that. I follow my heart to Teshima Island—because it is there, up ahead of me, on the island of my dream. I am following my heart because I haven't found it, then. I am searching for *mine* by following it?

It's hard to have a heart. I can't even say what it means clearly and distinctly.

Access to the archives is difficult. The island is served by modern transportation, but the journey will be challenging. I will fly to Tokyo, take a connecting flight or bullet train to the port city of Okayama, then a bus, taxi, or longish walk to the port, where I catch a ferry that takes me to an island where I transfer to a smaller ferry that delivers me to Teshima Island. Much time is spent waiting in ports or at stations. It is slow-going. Once on Teshima, I need a bus, bike, or car to reach the Teshima Museum from which I can walk to the archive. The path runs through a not dense but nevertheless dark forest. Where my day ends and where I spend the night remain unclear to me. The collection of hearts is found in a nondescript house tucked under some trees on a beach where the earth runs into the sea and dissolves.

It's a long way to go to look for a heart. Listening to mine might lead me to the edge of the world, and maybe over the edge. In my dreams, the island of hearts is perpetually lost in

September 1, 2008

## Les archives

the fog, surrounded by mist, as I see it on the screen of my computer.

It is by design that the place is "relatively hidden," Boltanski says, a sort of "lost island" (310). It's an almost timeless place and unworldly. The perfect place for dreams. A mythic island.

If Teshima is a time and place apart, going there is a ritual and Boltanski something like a preacher or shaman leading me through the dreamworld. He admits a fascination with religion, its forms, altars, votives, and so on, but also with the responsibility it can take for existential communications and forming our spirits. Josef Beuys is an avowed father. In times when much of the artworld is suspicious of religion, Boltanski is not afraid to say to an interviewer, "the artist is a preacher."[14] At a talk on Teshima, he is even more expansive about his religious vocation.

> What I am interested in now is creating a myth. I do not belong
> to any particular religious group or believe in any religion. I think,
> however, that there is a strong connection between religion and

art, and I feel that a museum is like a church in the present age. As we know, the process of looking for the key to the truth of something we cannot understand may be more meaningful than choosing the right key. . . . If I had been born in Africa, I would have been a shaman. If I had been born in Japan in the 19th century, I would have been a monk. I was born in France, however, in the 20th century, so I became an artist.[5]

There is a difference, though, Boltanski says, between the traditional believer or believer who adheres to a tradition, on one hand, and the artist, on the other, with a secular flock whom he ministers. That difference is, he says, "a monk might think he knows the answers" whereas the artist does not; for the artist, "what counts is to pose the question" (300). He might not be entirely right about the monk and his purported certainties, and the religions in which Boltanski says he does not believe might also cultivate an unknowing of answers, but about his own works he is clear: they lead us into the big, grand questions of human being, like a religion often does. Boltanski identifies some. "There are just five or six: the search for God, sex, death, the beauty of nature" (83). Also "suffering," which he later adds to the list (159). Without entering into an argument about whether he is right or not about that list and the items on it, what interests me is that, in his work, they are frequently posed by a beating heart. It is as if Boltanski were telling me that listening to your heart means accessing the big questions that condition being human—and also assuring me that his art will minister to those who take on those questions. A grand undertaking. Religious even?

It is becoming harder to find time and space in contemporary society for dreams such as his and mine. The business of life does not leave much of it left for taking on these questions, and the pleasures that consume us in our blissful consumption of culture-become-entertainment-and-information have crowded out our dreaming of them. Our absorption in a life become business and pleasure (business or pleasure) has left us oblivious to the need and neediness from which the dreaming comes. Boltanski describes his own feelings of alienation from such a world. "I feel a bit different and often shunned by the artworld," he says. "I feel that the reason for this, consciously or not, is the reference in my work to religion, Judeo-Christianity" (162), a reference that serves his heartfelt preoccupations, in particular, he goes on to say, his concern with suffering.

Because they are big, the questions posed by having a heart are not many, and they haven't changed much over time, Boltanski says. For an art that cares about them, "there is no such thing as progress, just an unfurling, artistic subjects have been the same always since the beginning of time" (83). Artists with Boltanski's religious vocation respond repeatedly to the same big questions, their answers making no progress except to bring us back to the source of the questions, the heart—largely because these questions don't have solutions that would put them behind us. All we can do is again and again remember to ask them. While each generation might outgrow previous ones by solving the small problems of life, none will outdistance its predecessor in answering the big questions that come from the chronic condition of having a heart. Progress is made by specialization. Specializing allows for small problems to be constituted and can make for expertise that solves them. Specialists specialize, after all, and so become the experts who solve our problems, and we make progress. But few to none specialize in big questions. For big questions, ones like suffering, awe in the face of beauty, the search for transcendence, life and death, generalists might be called for, and there is little recognition granted to them by our societies—not even by our learned societies, academies which have become too learned for that.

These big questions are what Boltanski's art is dedicated to addressing. I have called them matters of the heart. They are also questions that religious texts and authors, religious myths and rituals, have a history of addressing. At its best, I tell students, religion does not solve these questions of life and death; despite forms common today, religion is not morality or techno-science, which for the most part do claim to have solutions. At its best, religion provides a time and space where such questions can be admitted and so owned as constitutive of being human. The questions that come from the heart might be what religion has long admitted into our lives with its myths, rituals, and symbols, its stories, practices, and beliefs, but religion does not speak in compelling ways for many of us today. Because it is hard to have a heart, and because in a society like ours it can be even harder, there might be a need for secular priests who minister or shamans who guide us to the secular heart, helping us listen to it and find it. There might be a need for artists like Boltanski, in other words, and also teachers, professors, who take on that calling.

My dream of Teshima Island, a dream that borders on religious, was interrupted in July 2019, when I returned to Washington, DC, where I saw a show called *Manifesto: Art X Agency*. It was not a good place for someone who has lost it to look for a heart. The show was particularly painful to me at this moment in my life when, as a patient, "agency" feels a distant ideal and something of an accusation depreciating all the truth and reality, the facts of life, disclosed by listening to the heart of the patient I have become. It was as if it were telling me that my preoccupations of the past year were misguided and incorrect; that my absorption in matters of the heart, dreaming of finding mine on

Teshima, all that was insufficiently engaged and irresponsible—
irrelevant, maybe even indulgent. I needed to move on, it was
telling me, get over the big questions of my heart, and help "us"
make progress on the many problems we face today in our present actuality. It would probably also help me feel better to be
engaged and active, as my colleagues in cognitive and behavioral
science tell me the studies show.

What I needed was not a heart but a manifesto. Stop listening to what comes from the heart and answer the call of the manifesto. Join the cause. That's what the wall didactic shouted at me.

> The manifesto (a published declaration of principles or aims) has
> played a key role in the history of modern art. Starting with the
> *Manifesto of Futurism* in 1909, it has been the ideal form which
> artists have engaged with the political and social issues of the
> time. . . . [The final room of the exhibition] shows examples of
> how contemporary artistic practices have taken on the revolution-
> ary and critical impulses of the manifesto to address some of the
> key problems of our time, including gender and racial equality,
> nationalism and immigration, and the power of institutions.

Calling for a lucid, critical thinking that attends to the pressing
actualities of the world and all its problems, the manifesto urges
us to take action solving those problems, chiefly of a social and
political nature. Art is no exception, devotees of the manifesto
claim: it should engage social realities and itself be an intervention in the political realm where the key, defining problems of
our time are constituted and solved.

This was enough to shatter my dreams of Teshima Island.
The examples in the final room issued strong reminders, clar-
ion calls really, that the world was going to hell, that inequities
were rife, that xenophobic responses to others were toxic, that the

climate was no longer sustainable, that institutions were corrupt and where they weren't nobody trusted them or cared about them anyway. These were not just problems to study but problems to solve by engaged action committed to what the manifesto called for. What matters, then, is not the heart your work comes from or the heart that you put into it, the manifesto told me, but the cause to which you are committed and the results of actions undertaken in the name of that cause. To believers of the manifesto of art and agency, my dream of following my heart to Teshima Island must look like an escape, a distraction from the important political and social issues of my times, a flight from the things that really count in the real world. It probably also looks sentimental. They are not wrong. I should internalize those voices, make them part of an inner dialogue, and take the concerns seriously.

But still, I could not escape the sense that the work of *Manifesto: Art X Agency* lacked heart. Much of it did not seem to respond to anything other than the manifesto. I guess that was the point, but something seemed missing, the works felt hollow, as if nobody had put their heart into them. What seemed to matter is that the work come from confident belief in what the manifesto declared. That means idea before work of art and results in a work, as I saw at the show, that speaks to a mind or intellect, too often one that already knows what is being said to it since it already holds to the manifesto in its belief. Though it touched on important social issues, the work was not very touching—at least it didn't touch me, and not being touched, I wasn't moved, at all, to anything at all, action or otherwise. I just entertained ideas and not very enjoyably. In the end, it felt like the opposite of what the manifesto called for: a distraction not an engagement, one that did similar injustice to art by making work that appeared to me to be equally distracted from its calling.

Disappointed and even pained by what I saw and heard shouted to me at *Manifesto: Art X Agency*, I thought again of Boltanski. In an interview with Catherine Grenier, he is adamant that art is not about doing politics. Responding to her question about how the political events of May 1968 influenced his work, for instance, Boltanski says, "they had hardly any. . . . The climate surrounding May 68 had some impact on my work, but I was hardly politicized." He then continues to speak more programmatically: "When you are an artist, you must not be distracted and doing politics is a distraction. . . . For me politics is escapism. Like loving beautiful clothes or the excessive love of beautiful cars is escapism" (64–65).[6] Boltanski's ideal of the artist is austere and extreme, to be sure. He has also said, "we artists are not in the world, we're a little outside. We don't live anymore when we are artists."[7] Not of this world and seeming to have sacrificed what is important about life as we know it, Boltanski's artist resembles a priest or a desert monk with a religious vocation.

Many are puzzled by this seeming unworldliness and singular focus beyond the political and the social, including Grenier, who says to him in shock, "The actualities of the present world have no effect on your creation?" (65). But, as I left *Manifesto*, I took heart from my recollection of Boltanski's work. It was reassuring to recall a work of art that is confident about coming out of and going back into concerns that are not exhausted by the politically and socially effective. There is more to being human, more that is interesting about human being, more to talk about and to study, I hear Boltanski tell me. The artist with a priestly vocation can minister that excess by doing work that unveils realities that are real and pressing even if not of immediate political and social concern.

Where does that work come from? Boltanski says the heart. Take *Inventaires*, his collections of trivial, everyday objects belonging to people now dead who once lived in a small town whose name nobody even recognizes. Politically inconsequential, yes, but telling us of matters that matter. Where did it originate? According to Boltanski, in an idea that laid hold of his heart. "Dear Sirs," he wrote to the directors of some fifty museums, "An idea has seized hold of my heart. I would like to present all the objects possessed by someone . . ." (87). If we lose heart, are we exhausted by manifestos, on the one hand, and entertainment and consumption, on the other? All can be exhausting. I need to think my loves and concerns exceed those extremes. Boltanski's work gives cause to dream that they do.

Speaking more directly about the matters that seize hold of his heart, Boltanski says that he does work about "the poverty of humanity" or "the glory of mankind" (66). A press description goes so far as to say, "Christian Boltanski explores the themes of human life and death." What does that tell you about his work and particular works? It's so indeterminate and unspecific as to be about everything, so general as to be of no particular concern to anybody in particular. There is no apparent problem Boltanski cares about, no "actuality of the present world" with which it seems concerned, so how could his cares give rise to concerns that motivate any sort of meaningful action or work? What good is that?

That is the manifesto speaking, not my heart. Seen from the inverted perspective of Teshima Island, however, life and death and all the matters of the heart that come with its chronic condition do not appear to be problems. That's worth remembering. Life and death, love and hate, evil and moral paradox, suffering, all matters of the heart are big questions but not problems. It might be easier to stay focused on problems so that one can have solutions and know the answer. People respect you for that. But, I hear Boltanski telling me, listening to your heart is not a problem, questionable maybe and surely less convenient and more costly if it means going all the way to Teshima Island, but it's not a problem. I have been looking for someone to tell me that for a while now and not just tell me that but minister to the need to take on that chronic condition. Boltanski offers a myth that supports my vision, a ritual that gets me to a place dedicated to that lesson, and a shaman to guide me in my dream—for that's all it is, a dream.

One of the places Boltanski found hearts for his collection was the Grand Palais in Paris, where *Personnes* was installed as part of the Monumenta series in 2010.

*Personnes* is a transitional work in the collection of hearts leading to *Les archives du coeur*. "Heart" as an item collected was new, but collecting had long figured in Boltanski's work. In fact, it was what launched his career as an artist. Notable in this regard are the series of *Reconstitutions* (begun in 1970) and *Inventaires* (begun in 1973), displays of items belonging to persons, some dead, some alive. The inventory comprised the personal effects or objects that a person found herself with every day: toothbrush, coffeepot, bedstand, umbrella, pencils, eyeglasses, keys, letters, lockets, brooches . . . all the things I have in hand most of my time, the objects of my most immediate everyday concern, all the things or objects in which we invest ourselves collected and exhibited in boxes, tins or vitrines. They are not very interesting in and of themselves, tiny and insignificant, and Boltanski did nothing artistic to change or modify them, yet you are drawn in, you bend down and come close, magnify them in your close-up view. If it is to be more than junk, if these trivial, everyday objects become interesting and important, engaging and appealing, it is owing to the ardor or enthusiasm with which they are so lovingly collected and arranged by Boltanski, then correspondingly witnessed by me, the visitor. Whether or not you, the visitor, and he, the collector, put your heart into it makes all the difference. The work does not come from a manifesto.

In such collections, Boltanski appears to gather together what makes an individual that individual by showing the sum of her cares and concerns in the things where they materialize. The titles, *Inventaires* and *Reconstitutions*, suggest the collecting is a way to save the dead or absent individual, preserve her and present her as who she is, reconstitute her by listing, inventorying, the things of her everyday concern.

Matters are not that simple, however. While his work of collecting and archiving is frequently described as a struggle to save us from oblivion, Boltanski has a keen sense that it does not succeed. "Art is an attempt to stop death, the fleeting passage of time," Boltanski says. But, he continues,

> art is always a sort of failure, a combat you cannot win. You try to stop life, you see a beautiful sunset and you try to seize hold of it, but you cannot. Or you can try again each day to paint a portrait of your brother, you will not make him immortal, he will grow old, he will change. . . . Nothing can be preserved, but among some artists, you find a desire to play with that, to try to do it while knowing it is impossible. The work of archiving that I have been engaged in ever since the beginning, this will to keep a trace of it all, translates a desire of this kind, a desire to arrest death. (94–95)

The death that art stops appears at the heart of what it saves. "As soon as you try to freeze something, you kill it. My work with photography is connected to this. . . . Think of Magritte. If you take this pipe, for instance, and put it in a vitrine, it will no longer be a pipe but an image of a pipe" (86). Boltanski's collecting springs from a desire to stop what it has accepted cannot be stopped, death and loss. This unaccepting acceptance, this accepting of the unaccepted, takes form in the work of art, in which a hollow is made for the death it fights against.

*Inventaires* and *Reconstitutions* succeed, then, not because they let us see the individual in the collection of things, but because they make us sense her absence in the collection of all the things that present her. Collecting the personal effects, the achievements, or the papers of an individual—all that "teaches nothing about somebody." The person is not there, nobody is there. In fact, then, Boltanski's collections of personal effects constitute what he calls "a hollow portrait" (85). What is missing from the inventory? What is lacking in the hollow? The heart? Lost cause of those effects being personal and not just effects, the heart that has to be put into the hollow if the personal is to be more than just an effect but the living of a life?

The missing heart absent from the "hollow portraits" is found in *Personnes*, where that absence looms over us and becomes resoundingly clear in the ever-present sound beating throughout the Grand Palais.

The title of the show is apt. *Personnes* in French is both "people" or "persons" and "nobodies." *Personnes*, shirts, pants, sweaters, scarves, overcoats, hats and gloves, all the things with which we clothe ourselves are collected on the floor of the Grand Palais, a 13,500-square-meter exhibition space in a building originally constructed for the 1900 World's Fair. The clothing is of all sizes and colors, styles and seasons. It is displayed, as in *Inventaires* and *Reconstitutions* except without boxes and vitrines, in a grid of what resemble city blocks along hypothetical avenues. Those streets are dominated by a massive, ten-ton, more-than-thirty-foot-tall pile of similarly vacant clothes looming at the far end of the hall. Over that pile stands an enormous crane, continually picking up and dropping at random bucketsful of clothes of various sizes from the one mass piled up at the end. Before entering the city, visitors confront a wall of numbered boxes, rusty and dented, that obstructs their view and slows their motion. The boxes come from Boltanski's previous collections in the *Inventaires* series and *The Dead Swiss*. What the boxes contain is not known, but you quickly think of a morgue and boxes that hold cremains or personal effects. I think also of a vast impersonal library cataloging names and information, identity cards locked away, perhaps as part of a Nazi program of extermination.

Once beyond the wall, you are in a strange and foreign land, both city and cemetery, populated by *personnes*, at once people and nobodies, a land that feels full of nobodies and empty of persons who are there. "There is nobody here and yet the place is crowded," Laura Cumming writes for *The Guardian*. Amidst the piles and piles that crowd the place, you look for signs of life but find nothing. You might think of camps and encampments, of displaced persons or else extermination camps. Cumming describes it this way:

> Sixty-nine camps, but there are no tents and no living people, only thousands of old clothes lying face down on the floor. Is this where they fell or where they were laid? . . . You walk, you look, you search for evidence among the mildewed raincoats and threadbare denim. Here is a corduroy jacket, almost new, and a faded gabardine; there is a baby's knitted cardigan. They were young, they were old, they were not ready to die, poor departed souls who leave nothing behind but shucked garments.[8]

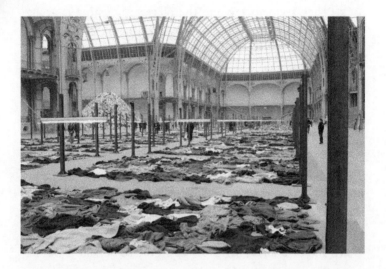

Whether murdered by others or exhausted by the effort of their own existence, the clothes show no signs of life. Hollow portraits. "Poor departed souls."

The presence of those departed souls is insistent. It looms over all of us—in the ambient sound of a heart, or hearts, beating throughout the Grand Palais. It comes from nowhere and from everywhere, but it is most decidedly not housed in the clothes where one wishes to find it. You cannot but sense, listen to, the omnipresent absence, the omniabsent presence—the lost heart found, the absent cause of the life of the dead effects lying on the floor.

It must be overwhelming to see piles of dead personal effects while hearing the most intimate sound of life pulsing outside them. Piles and piles of them, gathered into nothing like a living individual. We might remember somebody wearing something like that, but seeing them there on the floor in a pile, that memory does not arouse any joyful expectation of somebody returning with them on. "He is not here and won't be coming back," they seem to say like the places Augustine is accustomed to inhabiting with his now dead friend (see *Confessions* 4). The personal effects add up to no person—hollow portraits, the hollowness all the more insistent in that the heart that should enliven them, the heart where those concerns gather and weigh, is resoundingly not in them but outside.

Desolation and devastation hold sway over the entire place. If one has a heart, one is devastated, too. It's logical, the logic of the heart tells me I would resonate with it, that desolation would resonate in me, and I too would be devastated by its devastation.

That does not come from a manifesto but from the heart.

When I left *Manifesto: Art X Agency*, I did so because I was listening to my heart, but the believers in the manifesto do have a point: there are important social issues that need to be addressed politically. I would like to find a way to listen to my heart and not be irresponsible, to dream and not be deluded at the same time—in short, to be an agent *and* a heartfelt being.

Without speaking directly of present realities and historical actualities, Boltanski's work finds in me the heart to care about them. A heart that is neither irrelevant nor worldless? A heart that is worldless but therefore worldly relevant? Even if it is true that, as Grenier puts it, "the present actuality of the world has no effect on [Boltanski's] creation," even if he thinks doing politics is a distraction for an artist, escapism, it might also be the case that work in retreat from present actuality proves actually very relevant to the present and conveys its urgency. Tehching Hsieh has described how this might be. "I don't think art can change the world. But at least art can help us unveil life. I do have political awareness, but I am not a political artist. It is my reality that compels me to confront political issues. . . . I am inclined to observe the universal circumstances of human being instead of pointing to issues. The more I give a critical commentary on political powers, the less powerful my art will become."⁹ The power of Hsieh's art, he says, comes from the confrontation with reality, unveiling life so that we are made to inhabit our being and existence, our world and life, reality in short, where without "pointing to issues," the mattering of those issues is disclosed. Such a disclosure is heartfelt.

When the work finds the heart in you and you listen to it, as you can at Boltanski's *Personnes*, you are given to think of all the persons who are nobody (poor departed souls) and all the nobodies who are persons (the least of the earth). One's mind runs off to thoughts of Rwanda and Srebrenica, tsunami in India and earthquakes in Christchurch, children at Sandy Hook and Utøya, families on the borders of Syria and Xinjiang, and . . . and . . . and . . . the list goes sadly on. There are no explicit references to any of these places or people, however, no images drawn from these present actualities, no issues pointed to, and yet despite the absence of historically specific references and despite the absence of clear and distinct calls to mobilize, I am still given to think of each and all of them and more by the piles of clothing and the hearts beating.

Which is not so irrelevant or worldless. Listening to your heart might not be the escapism that the believers in the manifesto would have me believe.

The absence of explicit references to present actualities makes us take a step back from the prevailing imagery of the infotainment that so dominates our sensibility that we see and feel nothing. In the thoughtful spaces of Boltanski's retreat we might come to feel more deeply, think more sensibly, and maybe get to the heart of the matter. Are these different matters than the ones of political concern? Perhaps not. Perhaps it is that those matters now appear in the heart where they matter, where they are touching, where they touch us, and where the "real" world becomes really real. Perhaps reality is seen, not escaped, seen and

also felt, in the retreat from the real world to the retreat on Teshima Island or at the Grand Palais. The reality of things might
be such that we need a retreat from it, so that we can find the
heart to feel and feeling it, really be in it. Then it is not escapism
but reality clearly seen that calls for such a retreat from which it
becomes possible to engage the real world in a heartfelt way. The
greatness of Boltanski's work might be to heed that call. Only
from such retreats can real advances be made, and perhaps vic-
tories are even won by retreats like this.

Some, colleagues, critics, and others, will be suspicious of my
dream, the priestly vocation of the artist, the retreat that shelters
heartfelt thinking, feeling *personnes* in the heart, and so on. They
will call it "sentimental," among other things. It's a dreamworld,
a dream of a world, not a world, indeed an escape, they will still
insist, from the world into pure feeling, the misty, dreamy light of
a mythic island where I can be absorbed in my heart and matters
of the heart. Dreaming like this, I am given to feel but not act,
they will tell me. At best, that feeling is not just personal but feeling for others, feeling the pain of the world, feeling the social
and political concerns of the times, but even then, they will say,
feeling is not action, not even a guarantee of action. That's true. I
can be moved but not join the movement or even move at all.

But is sentimentality entirely bad? We might need the sentimental to help us dream, and we, at least I, need to have some
dreams if not of utopia at least of newtopia, especially these days
when I have lost heart. How bad is it to dream out of need? I have
tried to do so throughout this year or so of writing, maybe a bit
sentimentally, about the heart and what it feels like to have the
one I call mine.

So call it sentimental if you will, but sentimentality need not
be an insult. I have learned that in the course of this year finding

a heart to lose. Boltanski has given me some confidence in taking on the charge. Assuming it true that Boltanski's work is conceptual, as many would say, he shows me that not every concept need be heartless.[10] He embraces sentimentality, using as praise a term that is most often intended in his circles as derision. "My work has always been very sentimental," he says, "not very theoretical" (82). During an interview for *BOMB*, the interviewer points out that "so much of what has gone on in the West in terms of contemporary art has been just head," to which Boltanski responds, "yes, and to say an awful thing for myself, I am really happy if people cry a lot when they're looking at my work."[11] My work, he says, does not mean to be clever or intelligent, it does not want to keep you informed and up to date. It wants to make you cry. For that you just need to have a heart, or if you can't find the heart for it, let the work find the heart in you.

It's hard for me to have a heart today; everyday life as well as the professional circles I inhabit conspire against it. I am surely not the only one to find this to be so: disasters abound, in nature and society; suffering is everywhere; professional life ever more dependent on a cold, calculated regime in which you steel your heart for success; time always seems to be running out, in my day, for my homework, for the planet; and so on. Thinking about it in a heartfelt way can be overwhelming, devastating, a heartbreak every time. Boltanski gives me some confidence that my weakness for such thinking, sentimental though it might be, is a good thing. The best measure of its success or failure may very well be its ability to find the heart in us. Is that what makes it great: that it magnifies, celebrates and enhances, this weakness in us for a thinking that is not heartless; that it magnifies the thoughts that come from our heart and speak to our heart?

# THE END . . .

I am not the only one with sentimental dreams. People seem eager to go to Teshima Island and add their own to Boltanski's collection of hearts. One of the things that attracts us is the thought that our hearts will be saved, preserved for posterity in an archive. It is difficult to resist the lure of mine lasting forever. It is equally difficult to resist the attraction of having the hearts of others, my loved ones, ready and available, theirs too saved permanently in an archive. "You can go to this island and say, 'I want to listen to the heart of my grandmother," Boltanksi says,[1] and your desire will be satisfied. That is a dream come true, to have your own heart and that of the grandmother you hold in your heart, to have these hearts forever, saved forever. Your wishes will come true on this mythic island.

Is that what it's really about, however?

The facts are otherwise. "At the end of some years, all these hearts stored there now will be the hearts of the deceased, and this island will be something like 'the island of the dead'" (301). *Personnes*. A disappointing thought, sobering, a truth that can be disheartening. When you go there to listen to the heart of your grandmother, you will be listening to the heart that was her heart, a recording, an image. That's true of mine, too.

All that Boltanski said of *Inventaires* is also the case on Teshima Island. The work is not about saving things. The idea is that "it is impossible to preserve something." Nothing can be saved; persons cannot be revived. The recordings are not preserved heartbeats but reminders, a memory, keeping that loss. One day all that will remain of my heartbeat will be that memory, an image. Boltanski is lucidly aware of this. Speaking at the installation of his *Forêt des murmures*, he says:

> From the beginning of my creation, I kept trying to resist the idea
> of death as oblivion, but my attempts have failed. Instead, when
> I listen to the sound of the heartbeat of someone who already
> passed away, I feel the loss of the person. . . . I am at peace with
> the notion that someday, after my death, people will forget I ever
> existed. Even so, my wish is that people will keep coming to "Les
> Archives du Coeur" to record their own heartbeats, making it a
> new destination for pilgrims.

What am I really doing when I go to Teshima Island, then, if not making a memory of the death I will be? My life cannot be saved forever. What people will listen to when they go there is the heart that was my heart. A recording, an image. Listening to my heart as I make that recording today, I am already listening to the heart that was mine, the death I will be, in other words. My heart is the heart that will be the heart that was my heart. Those are the facts of the heart I call mine: the heart that will be the heart that was my heart is the heart my heart already is. My dream of Teshima Island a way of saying, impossibly, "I am dead."

Even the heart can be an image, a recording collected in boxes, electronic or otherwise, like the objects gathered together in the vitrines of Boltanski's *Inventaires*. Even the heart will be eventually only an image, like those objects in vitrines. That is what it is.

I don't want to see the heart added to the inventory of materials with which Boltanski works. I want it to be different from the clothes, toothbrushes, pencils, eyeglasses, and photographs. The most intimate of intimacies, the living of the life that houses it, I don't want to admit that it too can be archived like them. Why must my dream of Teshima Island lead back to his inventories?

The day always breaks, I wake up, and the dreams vanish. It can be disheartening even to think of mine being collectible like all the other collectibles, but the logic of the heart, the imperative that comes from it, tells me not to give up on the heart just because it can't be saved. People will keep coming to Teshima Island, as Boltanski says. Things, like life, like everything there is, that cannot be saved are not to be forgotten. I should not be oblivious to them. Don't give up on the heart just because it cannot be saved.

## . . . DREAM ON

*September 18, 2020.* One day my children will go to Teshima Island in the Japanese archipelago and visit *Les archives du coeur.* The archives were installed there in 2010 by the artist Christian Boltanski. A shrine as much as an archive, *Les archives du coeur* holds Boltanski's collection of heartbeats. Mine will be found there, and my children will listen to it and keep it close to theirs. They will make a day of it, an outing to Teshima Island to remember their father.

It's just a dream, remember, a sentimental dream.

I might go with them at some point, my son has said he will take me when he is an affluent engineer, but eventually they will go without me, for there will come a day when I cannot accompany them down that road or any other road. By that time, all that will remain of my heartbeat will be a memory. Not mine, but the memory deposited in the recording left in Boltanski's archive—and in those who remember, or are thoughtful enough, to visit the shrine. My heartbeat remains a memory, theirs.

By that time my heart will have become just a heart. I won't call it mine anymore. It will be mine only in their thoughts remembering it as "his." Without their memories it will be just a heart, in a collection like any other collectible, an item in a list. My heart lives on, has a future, thanks to them, thanks to their thoughtfulness in remembering and their remembering to be thoughtful. The future of my heart is in their memory.

I don't know what they will say or think while they are there or after they return home. I don't even know if they will go. My heart is in the hands of others, children, who might or might not remember to take on the weight. Dependency is like that, the future is like that, the future of my dependent heart.

It is a lot to ask of children and maybe even unfair of me: to have a heart that takes on the heart of their father. It's heavy, the responsibility of a generation for generations that are not their own, the responsibility of a generation for generating the future of a past that is mine not theirs. I don't expect it to be forever. I can't expect it of them. How will I fare with my own father's, my mother's?

The future I am dreaming of now is not one I will share with my children or they with me. It's a touching scene, a joyful one, imagining them going to Teshima to listen to my heart, but I won't partake of it. My children will listen to my heart beating in a time and place without me. I will not have a memory of this future, never be able to enjoy recollecting the truth of these images of love. It doesn't make me happy, therefore, this dream.

Its joy appears in sadness and tears, tears of joy. I can't hope to have that happiness, it exceeds my expectations.

What will happen to my heart? Where does it go when it leaves me like a pile of clothes and I put it in the hands of children? My heart might survive in their thoughtful memories, but I will never be able to say if that was or was not so. What my dream aims at is not being saved, not at eternity, but at being remembered, and memory does not last forever—at best three generations, maybe four these days. I can't ask for more and even that is a lot to ask. I don't expect to be remembered. Everything that is found will be lost eventually, even my heart.

# NOTES

## THE BEGINNING

1. From a profile by Calvin Tomkins, "The Turnaround Artist: Jeff Koons, Up from Banality," *New Yorker*, April 23, 2007.
2. Mark C. Taylor, *Recovering Place: Reflections on Stone Hill* (New York: Columbia University Press, 2014), 52. Subsequent quotations on 26, 3, 26, 110, and 33.
3. Heather Webb, *The Medieval Heart* (New Haven, CT: Yale University Press, 2010). My citations of Guido Calvacanti are found at 1, of Dante's *Vita Nuova* at 113 and 66. My citations of Dante's *Inferno* are from *The Divine Comedy*, trans. C. H. Sisson (New York: Oxford University Press, 1983).
4. Mark C. Taylor, *Field Notes from Elsewhere: Reflections on Dying and Living* (New York: Columbia University Press, 2009), 13.
5. Taylor, *Recovering Place*, 9.
6. Karen Green, *Bough Down* (Los Angeles: Siglio, 2013), 35.
7. I heard him tell the story in "Dario Robleto: Sculptor of Time and Loss," originally aired July 24, 2014, on Krista Tippett's radio show *On Being*.
8. Gallery guide to "Dario Robleto: The Boundary of Life Is Quietly Crossed" (August 16, 2014–January 4, 2015), commissioned by the Menil Collection University of Houston Cynthia Woods Mitchell Center for the Arts.

## AFTER THE FACT

1. Maylis de Kerangal, *The Heart*, trans. Sam Taylor (New York: Picador, 2016), 170.

2. Karl Ove Knausgaard, *My Struggle*, trans. Don Bartlett and Martin Aitken (Brooklyn: Archipelago, 2018), 6:183, 624.

3. Karl Ove Knausgaard, *My Struggle*, trans. Don Bartlett (New York: Farrar, Straus and Giroux, 2013), 1:3.

4. Quotations from *Thus Spoke Zarathustra* can be found in *The Portable Nietzsche*, ed. and trans. Walter Kaufmann (New York: Penguin, 1982), 353, 245, 352.

5. One of my favorite images of the spastic recoil in terror is the older sister, Claire, in Lars Von Trier's film *Melancholia*, riding here and there, all around, on an electric golf cart looking for a place to hide from the imminent arrival of Melancholia. Melancholia is the planet that will crash over all of us and destroy the entire world. When the truth is that the world will be destroyed, there is no place to hide. Looking for one is a denial of that truth and leads only to frantic, spastic movements of denial in search of what no amount of denial can make appear.

## I. THE HEART I CALL MINE

1. Eric Jager, *The Book of the Heart* (Chicago: University of Chicago Press, 2000), xx. Subsequent citations are found at 48 (citing Hraban Maur), 24 (citing Saint Ambrose), 116, 108, 111, 109, 110.

2. Jean-Jacques Rousseau, *Les confessions*, ed. Bernard Gagnebin and Marcel Raymond (Paris: Gallimard, 1973), 33–34. Translation mine.

3. Sandeep Jauhar, *Heart: A History* (New York: Farrar, Straus and Giroux, 2018), 72.

4. D. G. Melrose, B. Dreyer, H. Bentall, and J. Baker, "Elective Cardiac Arrest," *Lancet* 2, nos. 21–22 (July 2, 1955): 21–23.

5. See Mark S. Shiroishi, "Myocardial Protection: The Rebirth of Potassium-Based Cardioplegia," *Texas Heart Institute Journal* 26, no. 1 (November 1, 1999): 71–86.

6. A notable exception being images illustrating Proverbs 21:1, which reads in the King James Version, "The King's heart is in the hand of

the Lord." Other versions render it "the king's heart is like a waterway in the lord's hands."

7. On the design and implementation of the cardiac-pulmonary bypass machine, see John W. Hammon and Michael H. Hines, "Extracorporeal Circulation," in *Cardiac Surgery in the Adult* (5th ed.), ed. Lawrence H. Cohn and David H. Adams (New York: McGraw Hill, 2018), 299–346.

8. M. Salik Jahania, Roberta A. Gottlieb, and Robert M. Mentzer Jr., "Myocardial Protection," in Cohn and Adams, *Cardiac Surgery in the Adult*, 380.

9. I have been reading remarkable pages on birth in Louis Marin, *La voix excomuniée* (Paris: Galilée, 1981), including the sentence "I will be born" found in Stendhal, *Vie de Henri Brulard*.

10. Arthur Frank, *The Wounded Storyteller* (Chicago: University of Chicago Press, 1995), 23.

11. See Richard Shemin, MD, "Technique for Aortic Valve Replacement with Bioprosthetic and Prosthetic Valves," *Operative Techniques in Thoracic and Cardiovascular Surgery*, 5, no. 1 (November 2000), 251–53. Also "Aortic Valve Replacement with a Mechanical Cardiac Valve Prosthesis" and "Stented Bioprosthetic Aortic Valve Replacement," in Cohn and Adams, *Cardiac Surgery in the Adult*, 649–63 and 665–93.

12. "Elective Cardiac Arrest," in *Heart Surgery Classics*, ed. Larry W. Stephenson (Minneapolis: Adams, 1994), 158.

## 2. PRODUCING THE HEART

1. Stephenson and Baciewicz begin "History of Cardiac Surgery," the first chapter of Lawrence H. Cohn and David H. Adams, eds., *Cardiac Surgery in the Adult*, 5th ed. (New York: McGraw Hill, 2018), with Williams, writing about him: "This operation . . . is probably the first successful surgery involving a documented stab wound to the heart." But they note that Williams did not actually touch or put a stitch into the heart wound. This is why he is sometimes omitted from the history of heart surgery. Sandeep Jauhar does describe Williams's intervention in *Heart: A History* (New York: Farrar, Straus and Giroux, 2018), 61–65.

2. Jauhar, *Heart*, 65: "Credit for the first myocardial stitch resulting in survival belongs to Ludwig Rehn, a German surgeon, who, on September 9, 1896, sutured a two-centimeter laceration in the right ventricle of a twenty-two-year-old Frankfurt gardener." See also Stephenson and Baciewicz, "History of Cardiac Surgery," 3.

3. Jauhar dissents. He claims that in 1902, "Luther Hill became the first American surgeon to successfully suture a cardiac wound, in the left ventricle of a thirteen-year-old boy who had been stabbed five times." He also points to a report by Rehn in 1907 that there had been 120 surgeries on the heart with a forty percent success rate since the time he first put a stitch in a cardiac muscle (*Heart*, 68). James Forrester, by contrast, does not credit these claims or even mention Luther Hill, nor does the journalist Thomas Morris in *The Matter of the Heart: A History of the Heart in Eleven Surgeries* (New York: Thomas Dunne, 2018).

4. James Forrester, *The Heart Healers* (New York: St. Martin's, 2015), 54.

5. Morris, *The Matter of the Heart*.

6. Cited in Forrester, *The Heart Healers*, 32–33.

7. Forrester, *The Heart Healers*, 29–30.

8. "On Penetrating Cardiac Injuries and Cardiac Suturing," in *Heart Surgery Classics*, ed. Larry W. Stephenson (Minneapolis: Adams Publishing Group, 1994). The original can be found in *Archiv für klinische Chirurgie* 55 (1897):315–29.

9. Forrester says the success of its founding fathers depended on violating "an idea that stood sacrosanct for millennia, 'Do not touch the heart'" (*The Heart Healers*, 34).

10. Jauhar, *Heart: A History*, 62. One might suspect the brain to have been the last to be operated on, but Morris tells us that in 1884 Rickman Godlee removed a tumor from the skull of a man in London.

11. Ambrose Paré, *The workes of that famous chirurgion Ambrose Parey translated out of Latin and compared with the French* (London, 1665), 100.

12. Forrester cites Billroth on page 30 of *The Heart Healers*, Jauhar on pages 63 and 67 of *Heart*. Morris does, too. An important study of Billroth's reported remarks is provided by K. L. Schober in "The Quotation About the Heart: Comments on Theodor Billroth's Attitude Towards Cardiac Surgery," *The Thoracic and Cardiovascular Surgeon* 29, no. 3 (1981): 131–37. Schober notes that Billroth's remark is of uncertain date, often being dated much later, to the 1890s. Schober also

considers this remark in light of another, where Billroth says operations on the pericardium are a "prostitution" of surgery. This too has
been misdated. Put in the historical moment where Schober believes
it belongs, 1865, when the first edition of the textbook in which it
appears was published, rather than 1882, when a later edition was published, Billroth's remark appears prudent. In addition to being misdated, the citation is also taken out of context. Read in full, the passage adds "later generations may think otherwise." In context, then,
the remark comments on the current state of surgery, it is not a dictum
or legislative pronouncement. Schober then offers the hypothesis that
in fact Billroth never uttered the line attributed to him, that it was
mistakenly attributed to him on the basis of his written remark about
the prostitution of a pericardium suture.

13. Rudolf Haecker, "Experimentelle Studien zur Pathologie und Chirurgie des Herzens," *Archiv klinische Chirurgie* 84 (1907): 1035.

14. Jauhar, *Heart*, 65, 53. Galen, too, whose authority over medicine in the
west was almost unquestioned until the late Renaissance, claimed that
heart wounds were always fatal. Paré is cited by Morris in *The Matter
of the Heart*.

15. Paget's lines are cited in nearly all the historical literature I read and
even in some of the technical manuals and journals. See, for instance,
Forrester, *The Heart Healers*, 30; Mark S. Shiroishi, "Myocardial Pro-
tection: The Rebirth of Potassium-Based Cardioplegia," *Texas Heart
Institute Journal* 26, no. 1 (November 1, 1999): 82; and Cohn and Adams,
*Cardiac Surgery in the Adult*.

16. Jauhar, *Heart*, 67.

17. Mircea Eliade, *The Sacred and the Profane*, trans. Willard Trask (New
York: Harcourt Brace Jovanovich, 1959), 82, 89, 78, 80.

18. Dr. Francis Fontan, MD, who developed a procedure for rerouting circulation in bodies with hearts missing a right ventricle, conveys the
excitement of exploring the field: "In the late 1950's when I was a young
trainee in surgery, the field of congenital malformations was the most
attractive intellectually and the most demanding surgically, a field
where almost anything was to be discovered." Cited in Brian Doyle,
*The Wet Engine* (Corvallis: Oregon State University Press, 2012), 50.

19. See Bailey's report in "The Surgical Treatment of Mitral Stenosis,"
*Diseases of the Chest* 15 (1949): 377–97.

20. Forrester, *The Heart Healers*, 41. Frank Macek observes the novelty of addressing a chronic condition by repairing a valve: "Although valvular operations had been attempted nearly a quarter of a century prior [in the 1920s, first by Elliot Cutler and Claude Beck, then again by Henry Souttar], they were marked by limited success and therefore, infrequently attempted. Because of this, the realm of cardiac surgery remained largely restricted to repair of traumatic injuries and removal of foreign bodies." Bailey's operation on a mitral valve was preceded by T. Holmes Sellors's repair half a year earlier of a pulmonary valve by inserting a tenotomy knife through holding sutures in the right ventricle with a finger placed over the organ to gain "some sense of direction." See Macek's introduction to "Surgery of Pulmonary Stenosis: A Case in which the Pulmonary Valve was Successfully Divided," in Stephenson, *Heart Surgery Classics*, 51–53.

21. Forrester, *The Heart Healers*, 41–45.

22. C. Walt Lillehei, "Overview: Cardiopulmonary Bypass and Myocardial Protection," in Stephenson, *Heart Surgery Classics*, 121.

23. Cohn and Adams, *Cardiac Surgery in the Adult*, 6.

24. J. W. Kirklin, J. W. DuShane, R. T. Patrick, D. E. Donald, P. S. Hetzel, H. G. Harshbarger, and E. H. Wood, "Intracardiac Surgery with the Aid of a Mechanical Pump-Oxygenator System (Gibbon Type): Report of Eight Cases," in Stephenson, *Heart Surgery Classics*, 155.

25. Forrester, *The Heart Healers*, 52.

26. Forrester, *The Heart Healers*, 58–59.

27. Stephenson, *Heart Surgery Classics*, 158.

28. Stephenson, *Heart Surgery Classics*, 154.

29. Forrester, *The Heart Healers*, 73–74.

30. Stephenson, *Heart Surgery Classics*, 6.

31. See J .H. Gibbon, "The Development of the Heart-Lung Apparatus," *American Journal of Surgery* 135, no. 5 (May 1978): 608–19.

32. Forest Dodrill used a mechanical pump the year before "to substitute for the left ventricle for 50 minutes while a surgical procedure repaired the mitral valve," and he would use the same pump in a right heart bypass the following year when repairing a stenotic pulmonary valve. But Dodrill's pump did not include an oxygenator; it used the patient's lungs to oxygenate blood. What Gibbon and

Watson had designed, in contrast, allowed the entire heart to be stopped since it included an extracorporeal oxygenator as well. Stephenson, *Heart Surgery Classics*, 6.

33. "Valvular Surgery" in Stephenson, *Heart Surgery Classics*, 169.

34. One technique for installation is described by Richard Shemin, MD, "Technique for Aortic Valve Replacement with Bioprosthetic and Prosthetic Valves," *Operative Techniques in Thoracic and Cardiovascular Surgery* 5, no. 1 (November 2000): 251–53. Less detailed accounts of the procedure can also be found in Cohn and Adams, *Cardiac Surgery in the Adult*, chaps. 27 and 28.

35. As Hufnagel and colleagues recognize, "using techniques for deviation of the circulation, it would certainly be possible to place this valve in the ascending arch." C. A. Hufnagel W. P. Harvey, P. J. Rabil, and T. F. McDermott, "Surgical Correction of Aortic Insufficiency," *Surgery* 35 (1954): 673.

36. Brian Doyle does not agree with the claim that artistry has yielded to technique. Observing a heart operation, he writes, "Certainly there was vast technical skill at work . . . yet really the operation was a creative act." He then tells of an Australian surgeon who was observing with him and said, "any good surgeon could make a new heart out of an old one, sort of, but the interesting thing is no two surgeons would do it exactly the same way." Then speaking of the surgeon in action, the Australian says, "He's woidely [*sic*] disliked. But God gave him those hands. You can dislike a man, but you must be honest about his gifts, and God gave that man those hands" (Doyle, *The Wet Engine*, 74–75).

37. Stephenson, *Heart Surgery Classics*, 170.

## ON THE SLAUGHTER IN THE OPERATING ROOM IN HISTORY

1. Sandeep Jauhar, *Heart: A History* (New York: Farrar, Straus and Giroux, 2018), 85–86, 94.

2. G. W. F. Hegel, *Lectures on the Philosophy of History*, trans. J. Sibree (Milwaukee: American Home Library, 1902), 66.

3. James Forrester, *The Heart Healers* (New York: St. Martin's, 2015), 160, 162.

4. Stephen Pinker, *Enlightenment Now* (New York: Viking 2018), 39. Pinker is a bit too clean in his conscience, a bit heartless in his unhesitant celebration of progress, for me to commend the book unreservedly.

5. Brian Doyle, *The Wet Engine* (Corvallis: Oregon State University Press, 2012), 3. Subsequent citations are referenced parenthetically.

6. Arthur Frank, *The Wounded Storyteller: Body, Illness, and Ethics* (Chicago: University of Chicago Press, 2013), and *At the Will of the Body: Reflections on Illness* (Boston: Mariner, 2002).

7. Perhaps today, in a footnote: "that cold December day stays with me, the elderly mare 'which was otherwise to be killed as unfit for service,' the moist ground, the cawing ravens, the brass cannula in Hales' hand as he reaches into the heart of the hose, the wild eye of the horse, the grim look on the face of the stablehand as he sits on the horse's head, the leap of blood in the glass tube, the way Hales kneels and caresses the horse's jaw and she looks at him and he looks at her and what she is really, the horseness of her, her sweet salty spirit that never was before and will never be again, flies away" (Doyle, *The Wet Engine*, 16).

8. Forrester, *The Heart Healers*, 162; Jauhar, *Heart*, 85.

9. See Lawrence H. Cohn and David H. Adams, eds., *Cardiac Surgery in the Adult*, 5th ed. (New York: McGraw Hill, 2018), 134–36 and 751–59.

## 3. CONCEIVING THE HEART

1. Sandeep Jauhar, *Heart: A History* (New York: Farrar, Straus and Giroux, 2018), 51.

2. Cited in Margaret Lock, *Twice Dead: Organ Transplants and the Reinvention of Death* (Berkeley: University of California Press, 2002), 92.

3. Maylis de Kerangal, *The Heart*, trans. Sam Taylor (New York: Picador, 2016), 196, 31. Subsequent citations in this chapter are given parenthetically.

4. According to Margaret Lock, the phrase was invented by Thomas Starzl in the General Discussion that accompanied *Ethics in Medical Progress*, ed. G. E. W. Wolstenholme and Maeve O'Connor (Boston: Little, Brown, 1966). See Lock, *Twice Dead*, 94.

5. Lock, *Twice Dead*, 78.

6. Lock, *Twice Dead*, 91.

7. "Controversies in the Determination of Death: A White Paper of the President's Council on Bioethics" (December 2008), 28; Lock, *Twice Dead*, 60.

8. "With its special organs designed for movement, the heart, like some inner animal, [uses the rest of the body] as a dwelling-place." William Harvey, *Exercitatio Anatomica De Motu Cordis et Sanguinis in Animalibus*, trans. Chauncey Leake (Springfield, IL: Charles C. Thomas, 1928), 136.

9. William Harvey, *Exercitatio Anatomica De Motu Cordis et Sanguinis in Animalibus*, trans. Chauncey Leake (Springfield, IL: Charles C. Thomas, 1928), 136. Subsequent citations noted parenthetically.

10. Thomas Fuchs, *The Mechanization of the Heart: Harvey and Descartes*, trans. Marjorie Grene (Rochester, NY: University of Rochester Press, 2001). Subsequent citations noted parenthetically.

11. Others dispute the claim that Harvey was the *first* to conceive the heart as a pump and the motion of blood as a circle in the body. Bernat Hernandez points out that a Chinese medical manual more than 2,600 years old reports that the "blood in the body is pumped by the heart, completes a circle and never stops moving." See "How English Doctor William Harvey Upended What We Know About the Heart," *National Geographic*, February 13, 2018.

12. Heather Webb, *The Medieval Heart* (New Haven, CT: Yale University Press, 2010), 92.

## 4. LISTEN TO YOUR HEART

1. Paul Auster, *Ghosts* (New York: Penguin, 1987), 19–20.

2. "With its special organs designed for movement, the heart, like some inner animal, [uses the rest of the body] as a dwelling-place." William Harvey, *Exercitatio Anatomica De Motu Cordis et Sanguinis in Animalibus*, trans. Chauncey Leake (Springfield, IL: Charles C. Thomas, 1928), 136.

3. *The Philosophical Writings of Descartes*, ed. and trans. Dugald Murdoch, John Cottingham, and Robert Stoothof (Cambridge: Cambridge University Press, 1985), 3:134. Subsequent citations noted intertextually by volume number and page number.

4. Cited by Geoffrey Gorham in "The Harvey-Descartes Controversy," *Journal of the History of Ideas* 55, no. 2 (April 1994): 227. As Gorham notes, Harvey would claim later that blood, not the heart, contains the principle of motion.

5. On the confusion over systole and diastole and how the terms apply in Descartes, Harvey, and today, see Marjorie Grene, "The Heart and Blood: Descartes, Plemp, and Harvey," *Essays on the Philosophy and Science of René Descartes*, ed. Stephen Voss (Oxford: Oxford University Press, 1993), 324–36.

6. Cited in Martin Hägglund, *This Life: Secular Faith and Spiritual Freedom* (New York: Anchor Books, 2019), 63.

7. Brian Doyle, *The Wet Engine* (Corvallis: Oregon State University Press, 2012), 48.

## CURED OF THE HEART

1. Larry W. Stephenson, ed., *Heart Surgery Classics*, *Heart Surgery Classics* (Minneapolis: Adams, 1994), 170.

## 5. "UP WITH YOU NOW, COME ON, MY OLD HEART"

1. Friedrich Nietzsche, *The Gay Science*, trans. Walter Kauffman (New York: Vintage, 1974), §21.

2. In *The Portable Nietzsche*, ed. and trans. Walter Kauffman (New York: Penguin, 1977). Parenthetical references in the text are to this edition.

## 6. THE HEART'S IMPERATIVE

1. Citation from Stanley Cavell in *Senses of Walden* (Chicago: University of Chicago Press, 1981), 5. Citations from Thoreau in *Walden and Other Writings* (New York: Modern Library, 2000), 150, 92. Cavell references both passages from *Walden* on page 112 of *Senses of Walden*.

2. Thoreau, *Walden*, 117.

3. Adrian Heathfield and Tehching Hsieh, *Out of Now: The Lifeworks of Tehching Hsieh* (Cambridge, MA: Live Art Development Agency and MIT Press, 2009), 11. Subsequent citations noted parenthetically in my text.

4. Thomas A. Carlson, "With the World at Heart: Reading Cormac McCarthy's 'The Road' with Augustine and Heidegger," *Religion and Literature* 39, no. 3 (Autumn 2007): 54.

5. Peter Handke, "Essay on the Successful Day," in *The Jukebox and Other Essays on Storytelling*, trans. Ralph Manheim (New York: Farrar, Straus and Giroux, 1994), 147.

6. Stanley Cavell, *The Uncanniness of the Ordinary* (Stanford, CA: Stanford University Press, 1986), 117.

7. Maylis de Kerangal, *The Heart*, trans. Sam Taylor (New York: Picador, 2016) Citations can be found at 174–78.

8. Cormac McCarthy, *The Road* (New York: Vintage, 2006), 273.

9. The book: Thomas A. Carlson, *With the World at Heart: Studies in the Secular Today* (Chicago: University of Chicago Press, 2019). The article: "With the World at Heart." Citations are found in the latter at page 54, citing McCarthy, *The Road*, 220.

10. McCarthy, *The Road*, 53, 54.

11. Handke, "Essay on the Successful Day," 162.

12. Citations from De Kerangal, *The Heart*, 177–80.

## 7. PUT YOUR HEART IN IT

1. If "God" remains the name of faith's "object" or the name of what calls for faith, then what is called "God" introduces the absurd into everyday life. When Kierkegaard says that faith responds to "God," his call or command, he is saying something like faith leaps up in response to a call from I know not where to do what I do for reasons I don't know. Saying "God told me to do it" is equivalent, then, to saying "I don't know why I am doing it. I can't tell, and I certainly can't tell you others." God only knows, as we say, and he isn't telling.

2. Kim Levin, "Yves Klein's Leap Year," *ArtNews*, March 1, 2010, https://www.artnews.com/art-news/news/yves-kleins-leap-year-289/

3. Yves Klein, *Le dèpassement de la problématique de l'art* (La Louvière, Belgium: Éd. de Montbliart, 1959), 22.

4. From Yves Klein's *Sunday, November 27th, 1960, "Le journal d'un seul jour."*

5. Emmanuel Falque, *Métamorphose de la finitude* (Paris: Éditions du Cerf, 2004). The quotations are at 199, 200, and 201.

Deborah Sontag, "A Caged Man Breaks Out at Last," *New York Times*,
   February 25, 2009.
7. Ader's whereabouts are unknown. He disappeared in 1975, lost at sea
   attempting to cross the Atlantic Ocean in a sailboat. The boat, empty
   and floating bow down, was found in the waters 150 kilometers (93 mi.)
   off the shore of Ireland in April 1976. Ader is presumed to have died.
8. See Simon Critchley, *On Humour* (New York: Routledge, 2002),
   108–11.

## 8. HEARTFELT

1. "Monumenta 2010: Christian Boltanski," *Domus*, February 1, 2010,
   https://www.domusweb.it/en/art/2010/02/01/monumenta-2010
   -christian-boltanski.html.
2. Christian Boltanski and Catherine Grenier, *La vie possible de Christian
   Boltanski* (Paris: Editions du Seuil, 2007), 56. Subsequent citations are
   given in the text.
3. https://www.setouchiexplorer.com/les-archives-du-coeur/.
4. Irene Borger, "Christian Boltanski by Irene Borger," interview by Irene
   Borger, *BOMB* 26 (Winter 1989), https://bombmagazine.org/articles
   /1989/01/01/christian-boltanski/
5. The talk was held on July 18, 2016. It can be found at https://benesse
   -artsite.jp/en/story/20160729-652.html.
6. Grenier's interview with Boltanski was published in France in 2007.
7. Borger, "Christian Boltanski by Irene Borger."
8. Laura Cumming, "Christian Boltanski: Personnes," review of *Personnes*
   by Christian Boltanski, *The Guardian*, January 16, 2010, https://www
   .theguardian.com/artanddesign/2010/jan/17/christian-boltanski
   -personnnes-paris-review.
9. Adrian Heathfield and Tehching Hsieh, *Out of Now: The Lifeworks of
   Tehching Hsieh* (Cambridge, MA: Live Art Development Agency and
   MIT Press, 2009), 330.
10. An article in the popular journal *Wallpaper*, for instance, attributes his
    renown to having "introduced an emotional dimension to conceptual
    art at a time when most others denied it." https://www.mariangoodman
    .com/usr/documents/press/download_url/34/wallpaper-april-1
    -2018-.pdf.

11. Borger, "Christian Boltanski by Irene Borger."


## THE END . . .

1. Christian Boltanski and Catherine Grenier, *La vie possible de Christian Boltanski* (Paris: Editions du Seuil, 2007), 300–1. Subsequent citations are given in the text.

# ILLUSTRATION CREDITS

## THE BEGINNING

*Hanging Heart* by US artist Jeff Koons. Photograph by Emmanuel Dunand/ AFP via Getty Images.

Rendezvous With Jeff Koons in New York. Jeff Koons exhibition at the Metropolitan Museum of Art. Photograph by Hubert Fanthomme/Paris Match via Getty Images.

Mark C. Taylor, *Homage to Jeff Koons*. Photograph by Jeffrey Kosky.

Mark C. Taylor, *Hegel*. Photograph: Mark C. Taylor.

Mark C. Taylor, *neXus*. Photograph: Mark C. Taylor.

Mark C. Taylor, *Homage to Jeff Koons*. Photograph by Jeffrey Kosky.

Prosthetic valve. Photograph: Mediscan/Alamy Stock Photo.

Sphygmograph. Photograph: Alamy Stock Photo.

## CHAPTER I

Cardiac surgeons during a heart valve operation. Photo credit: Arctic-Images.

Open right atrium. Photo credit: ChaNaWiT.

John Calvin's seal of 1545 as found in C.-O. Viguet and D. Tissot, *Calvin d'après Calvin: Fragments extraits des oeuvres françaises du réformateur* (Geneva: Cherbuliez, 1864), 447. Image reproduced by kind permission of the H. Henry Meeter Center for Calvin Studies at Calvin University in Grand Rapids, Michigan.

John Calvin's seal of 1547 as found in C.-O. Viguet and D. Tissot, *Calvin d'après Calvin: Fragments extraits des oeuvres françaises du réformateur* (Geneva: Cherbuliez, 1864), 447. Image reproduced by kind permission of the H. Henry Meeter Center for Calvin Studies at Calvin University in Grand Rapids, Michigan.

Detail of a portrait by Pierre Woeriot (1566) as found in Emile Doumergue, *Iconographie Calvinienne* (Lausanne: G. Bridel, 1909), plates XIV and XV. Image reproduced by kind permission of the H. Henry Meeter Center for Calvin Studies at Calvin University in Grand Rapids, Michigan.

Heart surgery aortic valve replacement. Credit: Miralex.

## CHAPTER 2

A trifecta valve in its packaging. Photograph by Jeffrey Kosky.

## CHAPTER 6

Claire Kosky, *The book on Dad's Desk (#1)*. Credit: Claire Kosky.
Claire Kosky, *The book on Dad's Desk (#2)*. Credit: Claire Kosky.
Claire Kosky, *The book on Dad's Desk (#3)*. Credit: Claire Kosky.
Claire Kosky, *The book on Dad's Desk (#4)*. Credit: Claire Kosky.

## CHAPTER 7

Yves Klein (1928–1962) © ARS, NY. *Leap Into the Void*, 1960. Maker: Artistic Action by Yves Klein photographed by Harry Shunk (German, Reudnitz 1924–2006 New York (?)) and Janos (Jean) Kender (Hungarian, Pecs 1937–2009). Gelatin silver print. 25.9 × 20.0 cm (10 3/16 × 7 7/8 in.). Purchase, The Horace W. Goldsmith Foundation Gift, through Joyce and Robert Menschel, 1992 (1992.5112). Image copyright © The Metropolitan of Art. Image source: Art Resource, NY.

Shiva as the Lord of Dance. India, Tamil Nadu, circa 950–1000. Sculpture, copper alloy, 30 × 22.5 × 7 in. (76.20 × 57.15 × 17.78 cm). Anonymous gift (M.75.1). Los Angeles County Museum of Art, www.lacma.org.

Bas Jan Ader, *Broken Fall (Organic)*, Amsterdamse Bos, Holland, 1971/94. Silver gelatin print (framed). 18 × 25 in / 45.7 × 63.5 cm image size; 29.5 ×

36 × 1.5 in / 74.9 × 91.4 × 3.8 cm framed dimensions. Edition of 3. Credit: © 2024 Estate of Bas Jan Ader / Mary Sue Ader Andersen / Artists Rights Society (ARS), New York. Courtesy of Meliksetian | Briggs, Los Angeles.

## CHAPTER 8

*Oscar at Pulse (#1)*. Photograph by Jeffrey Kosky.

*Oscar at Pulse (#2)*. Photograph by Jeffrey Kosky.

*Oscar at Pulse (#3)*.Photograph by Jeffrey Kosky.

Screenshot (March 23, 2020).

Promenade at the Grand Palais, the World of Christian Boltanski, Paris, January 23, 2010. Photo by Jean-Pierre REY/Gamma-Rapho via Getty Images.

# INDEX

Paget, Stephen, 92, 102, 305

Paré, Ambroise, 90–92

passion, 56, 59, 232–50. *See also* heart, finding one's; heart, listening to one's; vocation

Pinker, Stephen, 108, 308

Plempius, 157

porosity, 14, 142–43. *See also* vulnerability

praise, 117, 119, 269, 271. *See also* prayer; thanksgiving

prayer, 59, 115–19, 178. *See also* contemplation; praise; thanksgiving

productivity, 12, 147, 149, 171, 175; industriousness, 175, 186–87

profane, 3, 86–95. *See also* disenchantment; secularity

progress, 105–20; progressophobia, 120. *See also* history, as progress; modernity; science

providence, 69, 119–20, 243. *See also amor fati*; Calvin, John; luck

purpose, 44, 93, 115, 157, 175–92, 226, 250. *See also* meaningfulness

recovery, xi, 7, 16–19, 145, 171, 177–82, 211, 238; convalescence, 176, 189, 191, 203; rehabilitation, 26. *See also* cure; healing; health; repair

redemption, 23, 110–11, 120, 162. *See also* compensation; sacrifice; salvation

Rehn, Ludwig, 86–92, 119, 304

religion, 7, 14, 92, 176, 277–80

resolve, 178–80, 197, 214–19; determination; hanging on; resoluteness; resolution. *See also* commitment

restlessness, 22, 37, 40, 58, 71, 135, 184, 236. *See also* Augustine of Hippo

ritual, 93, 277, 280, 285

Robleto, Dario, 28–32

Romano, Claude, 160

Rousseau, Jean-Jacques, 61–62

sacred, 2–4, 11, 18–23, 86, 92–95, 110. *See also* profane; sacrifice

sacrifice, 108–13. *See also* animals, in medical experimentation; compensation; redemption; slaughter

sadness, 113–18, 257, 273, 299. *See also* grief; happiness

salvation, 40, 296–99. *See also* redemption

science, 47–51, 105, 132, 281. *See also* disenchantment; modernity; progress; technology

secularity, 34, 58, 60; *saeculum*, 58, 73, 123; secularization, 73. *See also* condition, secular; death, secular; disenchantment; God, godlessness

self: -assertion, 151, 163; -discipline, 214; -harm, 246; -mastery, 68; -possession, 61, 77, 131, 151, 159–66, 171–72, 179; -reflection, 20; selfhood, 55, 160; -surrender, 69; -understanding, 63, 81, 85. *See also* authenticity; individuality; suicide